The Handbook of Disaster and Emergency Policies and Institutions

The Handbook of Disaster and Emergency Policies and Institutions

John Handmer and Stephen Dovers

EARTHSCAN

London • Sterling, VA

First published by Earthscan in the UK and USA in 2007

ISBN-13:   978-1-84407-359-7
Typeset by Safehouse Creative
Printed and bound in the UK by Antony Rowe, Chippenham
Cover design by Yvonne Booth

For a full list of publications please contact:

Earthscan
8–12 Camden High Street
London, NW1 0JH, UK
Tel: +44 (0)20 7387 8558
Fax: +44 (0)20 7387 8998
Email: earthinfo@earthscan.co.uk
Web: **www.earthscan.co.uk**

22883 Quicksilver Drive, Sterling, VA 20166-2012, USA

Earthscan publishes in association with the International Institute for Environment and
Development

A catalogue record for this book is available from the British Library

Library of Congress Cataloging-in-Publication Data

Handmer, John W.
    The handbook of disaster and emergency policies and institutions / John
Handmer and Stephen Dovers.
        p. cm.
    Includes bibliographical references.
    ISBN-13:   978-1-84407-359-7 (hardback)
    ISBN-10:   1-84407-359-9 (hardback)
    1. Emergency management. 2. Disaster relief. I. Dovers, Stephen II.
Title.
    HV551.2.H36 2007
    363.34'8–dc22

                                                                    2007024313

The paper used for this book is FSC-certified and
totally chlorine-free. FSC (the Forest Stewardship
Council) is an international network to promote
responsible management of the world's forests.

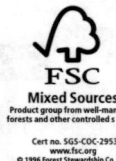

FSC
Mixed Sources
Product group from well-man
forests and other controlled s
Cert no. SGS-COC-2953
www.fsc.org
© 1996 Forest Stewardship Co

Contents

List of Figures, Tables and Boxes

Figures

Tables

Boxes

Acknowledgements

This book is a collaboration between an environmental policy specialist and an applied researcher in emergency management. We both owe debts to many people and organizations, and our thanks go to the many who are not named below. While we are collectively responsible for the scope and detail of this book, we have benefited enormously from countless interactions with colleagues, students, policy-makers and emergency managers from many parts of the world. In conceiving of and writing the book, we have, in many ways, drawn on Stephen Dovers' previous experience in writing *Environment and Sustainability Policy: Creation, Implementation, Evaluation* (2005, The Federation Press, Sydney), a project that itself had many debts.

Chas Keys, former deputy director general of the New South Wales (NSW) State Emergency Service, and Sarah Stuart-Black from the New Zealand Ministry of Civil Defence and Emergency Management, both encouraged the project, along with Rob West, Mike Fell, Camille Adamson and Alison Kuznets of Earthscan. A draft was reviewed with care by Tom Lowe of RMIT University's Centre for Risk and Community Safety, Chas Keys, and Paul Gabriel, policy director of Victoria's Office of the Emergency Services Commissioner. They provided many suggestions that we have tried to incorporate. Most importantly they were very positive about the project, and we hope the result does justice to their support. Ramona, Michele, Stuart and Emma had to endure in various ways the indirect impacts of a book-writing project.

We acknowledge and thank our many colleagues, both those at our universities and those practising what we write about in this volume. They provide inspiration and their challenging arguments help us refine ours. Both authors are members of the Australian Bushfire Cooperative Research Centre (CRC), a national research effort, which has introduced us to many new colleagues, problems and ways of thinking – and we are grateful for the support and opportunities the CRC has provided. Our work is made possible by the generous support of our home universities, the School of Mathematics and Geospatial Science at RMIT University and The Fenner School of Environment and Society at The Australian National University.

Work on the book was disrupted at times by the very emergencies we write about, although thankfully not ones of great tragedy. Hot dry conditions helped to ensure that New Year's Day 2006 was one of many extreme wildfire days in Victoria and kept one author busy as a volunteer fire-fighter through early 2006. Continuing drought and very hot weather saw an exceptionally early start to the fire season for the 2006 to 2007 Australian summer. Again, fire-fighters were busy, albeit largely on standby in the Mount Macedon area. A major urban interface fire during early October in Hobart meant unscheduled fieldwork. The other author experienced a summer and autumn of unusually intense storm activity, involving routine clearance of blocked and flooding drainage systems. One storm stalled the central business district (CBD) of Australia's capital city and damaged dozens of buildings at his university, including an overnight flooding of his computer. Such events focus the mind on trends influencing the incidence of emergencies in our lifestyles, in the Earth's climate and in policy styles seen in response.

In future, it is inevitable that societies will face more and more emergencies and disasters, and regrettably it seems similarly inevitable that the severity of these will increase in terms of impacts on people, livelihoods, economies and environments. Emergency management and disaster policy must rise to that challenge. This book seeks to provide focus and ideas on the broader policy and institutional settings that serve to enable or constrain what individuals, communities and emergency managers do to handle emergencies in the hope that their crucially important tasks can be made easier and more effective. This book is dedicated to those people.

John Handmer
Mount Macedon, Victoria
Australia

Stephen Dovers
Queanbeyan, New South Wales
Australia
July 2007

List of Acronyms and Abbreviations

ADPC	Asian Disaster Preparedness Centre
AFAC	Australasian Fire Authorities Council
BBC	British Broadcasting Corporation
CBD	central business district
CFU	community fire unit
CSIRO	Commonwealth Scientific and Industrial Research Organization
CUP	complex unbounded problem
DEFRA	UK Department for Environment, Food and Rural Affairs
DHS	US Department of Homeland Security
EMA	Emergency Management Australia
EMATrack	a database maintained by Emergency Management Australia
ERM	emergency risk management
FEMA	US Federal Emergency Management Agency
GBE	government business enterprise
GDP	gross domestic product
HDC	highly developed country
IFRC	International Federation of Red Cross and Red Crescent Societies
IPCC	Intergovernmental Panel on Climate Change
ISDR	International Strategy for Disaster Reduction
ICT	information and communication technology
km	kilometre
LDC	least developed country
MAFF	UK Ministry of Agriculture, Fisheries and Food
MCA	multi-criteria analysis
MDC	medium developed country
M&E	monitoring and evaluation
NGO	non-governmental organization
NPM	new public management
NSW	New South Wales
PNS	post-normal science
UCL	University College London
UK	United Kingdom
UN	United Nations
UNCED	United Nations Conference on Environment and Development

UNICEF   United Nations Children's Fund
UN–ISDR   United Nations International Strategy for Disaster Reduction
US   United States
WSSD   World Summit on Sustainable Development

Introduction:
The Context and Aims of this Book

It is too easy to be critical of emergency managers. In a major event, for them the stakes are high, with lives and economies at immediate risk, resources inadequate, and political and media scrutiny intense, interfering and unforgiving. Information will be inadequate, modelling ambiguous and rumours rife. Emergency management is often tested in public with immediate feedback, and a constituency dedicated to locating and punishing the blameworthy.

Disasters challenge societies and governments. They can undermine the legitimacy of government by creating apparent chaos and disruption, and by highlighting the weaknesses and limits of government. They can result in deaths and destruction, and disruption to every aspect of society. Poorer countries may find that 'the consequences of disasters erase years of development and take years to reverse' (Egeland, 2006). Such events also provide many opportunities, with the media, political and local constituencies generally endowing special status on those who show leadership and empathy with the affected. As short lived as this topicality and celebratory status may be, there are clear political benefits from many disasters. Paradoxically, the less visible process of strategic policy development and implementation for disaster reduction may carry little political reward, and its success in reducing the impacts of events that might otherwise become disasters may even result in budget cuts and reduced status and profile for those involved. This is because the media and political rewards are (not unnaturally) skewed towards the heroes of response, rather than towards strategic planners.

This all points to the desirability of developing policy that serves a number of aims – national and local; social, economic and environmental; focused on preparedness, response and long-term recovery – and that is flexible enough to cope with shifts in community and political priorities, while ensuring a high positive media and political profile. Such strategic policy is dependent on the suitability of the institutional settings within which policy is formulated, developed, implemented and monitored, and within which it evolves. Emergency management is the necessary and crucially important 'sharp' end of our societies' response to disasters, but is constrained or enabled by these policy and institutional settings. It is the intent of this book to contribute to emergency management by focusing on what we believe to be those overlooked policy and institutional settings. Emergency management and disaster policy is in a state of change and reflection, and we hope to contribute, critically and constructively, to that process of change and improvement.

The importance of thinking more broadly about disasters and emergencies has been recognized by many for some time. The doyen of hazard researchers, Gilbert White (1945), among others, has argued for policy and approaches that tackle human systems, as well as nature:

> It has become common in scientific as well as popular literature to consider floods as great natural adversaries ... to overpower... This simple and prevailing view neglects ... the possible feasibility of other forms of adjustment.

To fulfil the intent of White's instruction, we approach the topic of disasters and emergencies in a different manner than most other literature. The aim is to consider disasters as strategic policy and institutional challenges that demand 'increasing political space' (UN-ISDR, 2004)), and not just as events that impose themselves on our communities. This requires an understanding of:

- the nature of disasters as a phenomenon arising at the intersection of closely interdependent human and natural systems; and
- the nature of public policy and human institutions as the primary means whereby societies frame common problems and generate responses to those problems.

This book

Chapter 1 sets the scene by surveying the nature of disasters, emergencies, risks and hazards, and trends in emergency management. Selected 'vignettes' – brief case studies – are used to illustrate the major themes pursued in the book. Chapter 2 draws key insights from the fields of public policy and institutional design. We propose that the disasters and emergencies field has not benefited sufficiently from traditional policy and institutional thinking and seek to remedy that deficiency. Core terms and concepts describing policy and institutions are defined.

Chapter 3 brings together an understanding of the nature of disasters and the nature of policy and institutional systems, and constructs a framework for describing, analysing and prescribing disaster policy. This framework melds an extended emergency risk management model and a detailed policy cycle model, seeking to profit from and integrate the insights of both traditions of thought. The main elements of this framework are used to organize the remainder of the book, paying more attention to what comes before and after a disaster event than to the traditional focus on immediate response.

Chapter 4 deals with ownership of the problem of disasters, their political context, definitions and roles of different communities, and the nature of public participation and communication. Chapter 5 outlines how we frame the policy problem of disasters and emergencies, and the attributes of disasters that characterize them as policy problems and that shape the imperatives for societal response. Chapter 6 explores policy choice and implementation, and Chapter 7 details the issue of learning from experience and improving policy and institutional capacities over time – arguably the most critical aspects of all. Chapter 8 surveys the challenges and opportunities for establishing institutional settings more conducive to understanding, preparing for, responding to and learning from disasters and emergencies. In Chapter 9, we set out the main challenges for the future.

The book uses numerous illustrative examples of the good and the bad of emergency management and disaster policy, but does not include detailed worked case studies. Part of the reason is to keep the book short and accessible. But the key reason is that the literature, both formal and grey, is replete with detailed retrospectives of specific disaster events and the way in which they have been impressively or poorly conceived and handled (we refer to such studies and their insights). The point of this book, however, is to draw broader lessons – both cautionary and positive – from across the field in order to inform policy and institutional responses.

We have consciously avoided setting out a comprehensive bibliography. Instead, our intention is to provide a guide to further reading and material for those interested; nevertheless, the set of references is large. The list below is aimed more at the policy and cross-disciplinary reader than the specialist. The literature is very large and any small list will be very partial and fails to catalogue important contributors. Interested readers should also examine recent issues of some of the journals listed below to gain a better picture of contemporary thinking. As a general starting point, the following are suggested: *At Risk* (Wisner et al, 2004 – about vulnerability); *Know Risk* (UN-ISDR, 2005 – numerous examples of risk management); *Crucibles of Disasters: Megacities* (Ken Mitchell, 1999 – case studies of the vulnerability of large cities); *Disasters by Design* (Mileti, 1999 – current state of US research and practice; it attempts to blend disaster management with sustainable development and lists references in a wide range of disaster-related areas); *Environmental Management and Governance* is one of several policy-related volumes by Peter May and Ray Burby (May et al, 1996); work by Tom Drabek has concentrated on the practice of emergency management (e.g. Drabek and Hoetmer, 1991); while material on the economics of disaster and disaster policy is introduced in the World Bank's volume *Understanding the Economic and Financial Impacts of Natural Disasters* (Benson and Clay, 2004), *Disaster Loss Assessment Guidelines* (Handmer et al, 2002) and advice from the websites of the US Federal Emergency Management Agency (FEMA) (see below) and the UK's Flood Hazard Research Centre.

Journals in the field include *International Journal of Mass Emergencies and Disasters*, with an emphasis on sociology; *Contingencies and Crisis Management*, which comes from a management and public administration perspective; *Natural Hazards*, which emphasizes natural phenomena; the more people-centred *Environmental Hazards* and *Global Environmental Change*; *Natural Hazards Review*, a wide-ranging journal from the US engineering society; and *Society and Natural Resources*, which explores societal aspects of natural resource management. Journals serving the field directly include the *Australian Journal of Emergency Management*; the journal *Disaster Prevention and Management* and the journal *Disasters* (which is more oriented towards developing countries), in addition to many journals of a trade rather than academic nature. Specialist journals from all fields and from practice, such as *Risk Analysis*, *Water Resources Research*, *International Journal of Wildland Fire*, and many publications from natural resource management contain articles of value for emergency management. Sources more oriented towards practice include the *Emergency Management Australia (EMA) Handbook* series (www.ema.gov.au) and equivalent material from FEMA (www.fema.gov). Other sources include key organizations and their websites, such as EMA (www.ema.gov.au); United Nations International Strategy for Disaster Reduction (UN–ISDR, www.unisdr.org); the Hazards Center at the University of Colorado, Boulder, US (www.colorado.edu/hazards); the Asian Disaster Preparedness Centre (ADPC, www.adpc.net/), Bangkok, Thailand; and the Benfield UCL Hazard Research Centre at University College London, UK (www. benfieldhrc.org/).

Part I

Constructing the Problem

1

The Nature of Emergencies
and Disasters

Disasters, even if not large, are treated to intense media coverage with the consequent need for political involvement and public sympathy. But the disaster is almost always treated as an 'event', with media interest moving quickly to the next issue. Those affected, however, may find that the impacts are long lasting and extend well beyond the apparently affected area. Our aim in this book is to provide a framework to help shift the focus away from the event and towards longer-term thinking about the disaster process, including issues such as vulnerability, resilience, preparedness and recovery. This chapter sets out the basis for our approach in terms of contemporary thinking about disasters, their definition, trends and underlying causes, drawing on a broad characterization of the field and on some brief 'vignette' case studies.

We might argue with the statistics suggesting that the worldwide toll from disasters is escalating; but there is no argument that the impact of disasters on people's thinking and on the political agenda is much higher now than a few years ago. The Asian tsunami, Hurricane Katrina, heat waves in Europe, infrastructure failures in Australia and the US, transportation failures in Sweden and Indonesia, earthquakes in Pakistan, among many other events of every kind – and far more less or known ones – remind us of the limits of prevention, and the political and human costs of inadequate disaster response and recovery planning. Most of all, we are becoming aware of a shortage of longer-term strategic thinking and policy.

There are 90 million more human beings every year, and our societies and economies grow ever more complex and interdependent. The co-location of dense human settlements with potentially devastating natural and technological hazards suggests that we should expect more disasters, or at least more events that have the potential for disaster if not properly handled. The number of humans who exist in day-to-day survival mode, if not the proportion of the total population, appears to be increasing and is probably about half of all humanity – defined as those surviving on less than US$2 a day (UNDP, 2005) or who live in the 60 or so countries currently directly affected by warfare or violence. Such people have very limited capacity for disaster preparedness or recovery – their resources are inadequate for even their daily needs. This does not mean that people and their communities are not highly resourceful, but certainly their vulnerability to disruption is exacerbated.

Trends underlying increasing exposure and vulnerability may be exacerbated by the now near-universal use of risk analysis and management in decision-making across all areas of society as part of regulatory, commercial and management processes. Risk now occupies a central place in thinking about contemporary society, as illustrated by the work of the social theorists Beck (1992) and Giddens (2000), who argue that modern society is better understood in terms of risk rather than, for example, class. Risk occupies a key position in policy debates. Among other things, this acknowledges explicitly that most aspects of our lives are filled with uncertainty. However, almost every aspect of the risk concept is hotly contested. Potential problems for risk-based disaster management are that much attention can go to the trivial but easily measured or conceptualized, while, paradoxically, the process may also show that the risk of exotic animal disease, import of food produced with particular chemicals or escape of contaminants is low – and therefore acceptable. Acceptable risk is the 'residual' or remaining risk. In our context, 'acceptable' means that emergency managers, usually without consultation, will be responsible for dealing with the residual risk, effectively removing it from public debate. The implication is that acceptance of a risk, and the benefits that this may bring, is traded off (usually implicitly) against sound emergency management.

What are the essential components of a 'disaster' or 'emergency', and what constitutes 'vulnerability'? The field, like all others, has its own jargon. The question 'What is a disaster?' is the subject of three recent books, which examine the topic primarily from a research perspective (Quarantelli, 1998; Stallings, 2002; Rodriguez et al, 2006). Agencies and statutes also set out their definitions; but often it is the media who seem to have the power to declare an event or situation a 'disaster'. Charles Fritz (1961, p655) was possibly the first to articulate a definition in the research and policy literature. Disasters are:

> ... uncontrollable events that are concentrated in time or space, in which a society ... undergoes severe danger and incurs such losses ... that the social structure is disrupted and the fulfilment of all or some of the essential functions ... is prevented.

Today, we may have to accept that disasters are not capable of precise definition, especially given that we increasingly recognize that disasters may be complex in their genesis and create unexpected additional disasters as they proceed. No matter what the arguments of intellectuals or policy-makers are, the global media, epitomized by CNN, is likely to be the ultimate definer of 'disaster'.

Disasters are subject to numerous definitions: to an investment bank, they mark an investment opportunity in the same genre as investing in shares; they are research opportunities; and the livelihoods of many non-governmental organizations (NGOs) and professionals are built on them. To governments, disasters offer the opportunity to legitimize themselves, to parade their power by mobilizing resources, and to empathize with the victims by offering sympathy and assistance. Seen like this, disasters are social, political or economic phenomena, not visitations by some force external to human control or as a result of calculated engineering risk.

Overview of disaster trends

The global re-insurer Munich Re (2006, p48) observes that, since the 1950s, there has been a threefold increase in major natural disasters, an eightfold increase in losses from such events and a 15-fold increase in the losses carried by insurers. The peak year was 1995, at US$190 billion, or 0.7 per cent of global gross domestic product (GDP). This trend probably reflects the social trends set out below, as well as the global spread of insurance, rather than changes in the global environment (although climate change is certainly implicated). During the 1990s, disasters resulted in a global average each year of 75,250 deaths and 211 million people affected (Walter, 2001). These figures apply to all disasters other than warfare. These figures refer overwhelmingly to climatic hazards, with 90 per cent of the deaths from climatic agents.

Most of the human impact of natural disasters is in the developing world, as shown by the following figures illustrating the dramatic difference between rich and poor countries (IFRC, 2001 – from the IFRC database of 2557 disasters from 1991 to 2000):

- highly developed countries (HDCs): 22.5 deaths per disaster;
- countries with a medium level of development (MDCs): 145 deaths per disaster;
- least developed countries (LDCs): 1052 deaths per disaster.

It has been conventional wisdom that while developing countries bear the brunt of human losses from natural disasters, developed countries suffer more economically. While this may be the case in terms of gross total dollar cost, the poorer the country, the greater the proportional impact on national economies and development progress. Some well-known examples show this clearly:

- Hurricane Mitch (Honduras), 1998: 75 per cent of GDP;
- earthquake in Turkey, 1999: 7 to 9 per cent of GDP;
- Hurricane Andrew (US), 1992: <1 per cent of GDP.

Hazards are clearly a vitally important issue for poor countries, even if they are not reflected in budgetary or public-sector arrangements. It is to be expected that small countries would be more affected by a single hazard event than a large country since a single event could affect much of their territory and, thus, their infrastructure, productive capacity and human population. However, this explains only part of the variation in impact set out above. Many developing countries find that their hopes for development are severely constrained by natural hazards since survival and urgent daily priorities effectively undermine strategic disaster reduction policy. Some countries' abilities may also be constrained by internal conflict, weak institutions or other social or economic problems. Similar issues can arise for poorer regions of otherwise wealthy countries.

Emergency and disaster institutions

Emergency and disaster-related institutions and policy processes were not developed for the broader challenge of longer-term strategic policy development, but for effective *response*, and occasionally for *prevention*, emphasizing events well defined in space and time. For planning and response purposes, disasters are seen to affect a specified area for a specified time. These boundaries are generally defined in administrative terms as required by jurisdictional boundaries and budgets. Yet, many types of disasters have very long-lasting impacts, at least on some sections of society, and may have a near global reach. As critically important as the dominant bounded approach to disasters is (saving lives and protecting assets), ignoring broader policy and institutional settings creates a problem frame and response approach to the threat of disasters that can easily become reactive and less strategic.

Nevertheless, there have been attempts to broaden the scope of emergency management and to develop more strategic approaches and capacities. One attempt to broaden the approach to emergency management has been through the introduction of a risk-based framework and approach, known in Australia and New Zealand as Emergency Risk Management (ERM), based on the generic Australian–New Zealand Risk Management Standard (Standards Australia, 2004), which has become a model framework in the field. ERM is not a substitute for the policy process, although on paper (if less in actual practice) it contains some of the essential attributes of policy development and implementation. It sets out a process for guiding implementation of societal goals that are established elsewhere. An extended version of this framework is developed and connected to longer-term policy challenges in Chapter 3. The ERM approach offers a broad view of risk and the required response by spreading attention away from simply the event itself to include more explicit consideration of what is at risk, the context of emergencies and disasters, and consultation and communication.

This book proposes that such a broader view is required – but is too often missing – due to the underlying nature of disasters and emergencies, where phenomena with highly complex causes and effects exist well before and after specific events.

Our focus is primarily on levels 1 to 4a, as illustrated in Table 1.1, albeit with recurring reference to levels 4b and 5. This does not in any way discount the critical importance of the latter, but rather that we see a needed contribution in the policy and institutional dimensions of emergencies and disasters so that the more immediate ways in which we conceive of and respond to disasters can be enabled, and not constrained, by the policy processes and institutional settings within which emergency management operates. If levels 1 to 3, in particular (the negotiation of social goals, the policy and institutional environment, and the directions to emergency managers and communities issued from them), are imperfect, then emergency management is constrained. At best, responses to disasters will be inefficient, resources will be squandered, and cycles of blame will occur. At worst, lives will be lost and communities devastated, when the outcome could have been better.

Table 1.1 *Hierarchy of activities in emergencies and disasters*

Level	What (is done)? Who (does it)? How (do they do it)?
1 Social goals	• Negotiation of what is valued; expression (at least partially) of the goals of society. • Political system, executive, voting population, policy communities, epistemic communities, media. • Highly variable within political and institutional traditions, rules and styles.
2 Institutional systems and policy processes	• The 'rules of the game' and processes through which social goals are translated into action (or not). • Political system, governments, policy communities, epistemic communities. • Highly variable over time, jurisdictions and issues, but within political and institutional traditions, rules and styles.
3 Policy objectives	• The more precise targets and goals expressed in formal policy statements. • Largely the role of governments in various kinds of partnerships with non-government interests.
4a Policy implementation in the public sphere	• Design and implementation of policy programmes and instruments; monitoring and evaluation of these. • Government organizations/agencies and their partners (industry and community). • Through various strategies involving resources, statutory authority, information provision, etc., depending on context, instruments used, etc.
4b Policy implementation in the private sphere	• Provide infrastructure, services, insurance, etc. within regulatory and market settings relevant to preparedness, response and recovery. • Private firms, consultants, sole operators (e.g. trades people). Independently, in industry associations or contracted by governments. • In all the above, and also as individuals, households, and informal or formal community groupings.
5 Emergency management	• Preparedness for and response to events. • Emergency management sector and industry; key partners and related sectors (health, security, local communities, etc.). • Professionalized; highly responsive and rapidly changing in the face of events, policy shifts, community preferences, the media, etc.

Note: for definitions of policy-related terms, see Chapter 2.

The nature of disasters and emergencies: Cause and effect

The causes of impacts in, say, a flood can be explored by examining much more than the hydrological event itself. Vulnerability in this case might be defined by land-use planning or its absence, which allows settlement in hazardous areas; poverty that leaves little choice but to settle in flood-prone areas and in unsafe structures; inadequate transport and other infrastructure; poor educational and communication provision; and other factors. This connects with the long history of social vulnerability – the 'root causes' discussed in some disaster literature – and the complex social, economic and political interactions within communities, and between communities and the natural environment and other sources of hazards. Vulnerability may be much more a socially and politically constructed phenomenon than one determined by proximity to a source of natural hazard. If policy is to be strategic, and if institutional settings are to increase resilience and avoidance of impacts, then a focus on the 'event' alone may save lives and property, but will always be reactive and is unlikely to improve resilience. The *underlying causes of vulnerability* should be a target for disaster policy.

Disaster events themselves are not always clear and recognizable. The agent of disaster may be invisible, and there may be contamination rather than, or in addition to, more tangible and instant damage, as in New Orleans following Hurricane Katrina. Where there is contamination, it may be difficult to measure or identify until much later: the problem may be unbounded in time and space, with impacts persisting for decades. Often there is a clear beginning (but often not), and the problem may continue for generations (as in the Chelyabinsk area in Russia, following the nuclear accidents of the late 1950s), with contaminated soil and water, or irreversible change to economies, communities or ecosystems. Climate change, ozone depletion and biodiversity loss are universally seen as global environmental change issues; but many lower profile issues have international dimensions. This situation may occur, for example, through the pursuit of compensation in different jurisdictions than that of the event (e.g. the chemical accident at Bhopal), through expansion of regulations or best practice globally (e.g. transport, nuclear energy, dam safety and industrial accidents), through government and non-government aid, or by relocating activities banned in one jurisdiction to another.

Compensation is another key issue. Not all events may be compensated for or insured against. The global insurance industry talks of 'mega-perils', which may be unbounded. Insurers have never insured against radiation and are increasingly concerned about natural hazards and global environmental change. The industry is also concerned with more traditional events that are clearly bounded, but very expensive. These include major earthquakes in wealthy areas or large-scale natural events, with the US insurance industry, for example, gradually restricting cover for wildfire and hurricanes. With the exception of the UK, commercially available flood insurance is very limited. The insurance industry refers to – as does Beck (1992) – an uninsured future.

There is a widely held perception that there are now more disasters because of the increasing number of climate extremes or severe climatic events, resulting from shifts in global climate and other processes (Steffen et al, 2004). This appears to be the perception in Europe following a series of severe storms, floods and heat waves through the late 1980s, 1990s and into the 21st century. Yet, this is only part of the story. The evidence set out above concerning the global distribution of disaster losses suggests that even if there were fewer climatic extremes, we would, nevertheless, be seeing increasing losses. This is because social, economic and political factors, as well as our use of technology, are crucial to vulnerability and our ability to adapt. Climate and its manifestation through weather is an important contributor; but it is only one factor. The factors that appear to be important explanations of why climatic disasters are increasing are now identified – it is these factors that are most amenable to policy responses.

Knowledge and attitudes

Increasingly complete and sophisticated data may contribute to the size of the list of disasters and emergencies. Certainly, this is likely to be the case for smaller emergencies where data have, in the past, been at best erratic. However, major disasters have long attracted global media coverage, so the difference in the number of major events simply because we have become better at recording them is likely to be small. How we record and note them may have more influence. As insurance coverage spreads, for example, economic estimates of the cost of disasters can change our views on their impacts. Live media coverage and increasing international networks heighten awareness of distant events, and if the global media declares an event a 'disaster', it is difficult for politicians and civil society not to concur.

The impact of knowledge and attitudes is far greater in terms of our understanding of disaster potential. As our knowledge of the physical and social processes underlying disasters grows, so, it seems, does the potential for disaster. It is likely that the greatest influence is our changing attitudes to risk and danger – best seen through the proliferation of health and safety-related regulations, especially in more litigious societies, and our appreciation of vulnerability. It can seem that many people would like zero risk and seek compensation when this is not achieved. Perhaps more importantly, there may be intense interest – paranoia even – about the possibility of disaster. This could turn into an advantage if the attitude can be harnessed by emergency and disaster managers for long-term policy objectives, but is far less constructive if harnessed for other political reasons.

More usually, though, knowledge, awareness and sensitivity to disaster are heightened and widely sought only briefly following a major event. An inability to maintain attention over longer periods is anathema to the strategic development of policy and institutional responses.

Increasing frequency of climatic extremes

The evidence for increasing frequency of climatic extremes is mixed. That said, the Intergovernmental Panel on Climate Change (IPCC) represents the largest concentration of sustained scientific effort in history. Their recent report stated that 'evidence of global warming is now unequivocal' (IPCC, 2007). The impacts of warming are clearly visible in polar regions, and many research groups argue that some impacts are visible globally through an increase in extreme hot weather. Heat waves tend not to have major obvious economic impacts, but may result in massive loss of life. Warmer winters, fewer frosts and changed rainfall patterns have impacts on biodiversity and agriculture that may not be as media friendly, but may undermine local economies. Climatic extremes and climate change do not by themselves result in disaster: it is the interaction of climate through weather with human activity or assets that can produce disaster. The impacts are likely to be greatest in areas dependent on farming, especially subsistence agriculture. Studies of future flood loss in south-east England show that climate change would account for about 20 per cent of the increase in expected economic loss by 2020: the main factors were increased wealth and exposure (Foresight, 2004). Human exposure and vulnerability to disasters also increase with rising population.

Increase in world population, with most increase in poorer areas

All other things being equal, with higher populations any given event affects more people. Most population increase is in poor countries that are disproportionately affected by climatic hazards. In addition, many newly occupied areas were previously left vacant precisely because they are hazardous, especially on the fringes of (or in) poorly built infill in ever growing urban areas. This is best seen in areas prone to flooding, landslides and industrial pollution, now occupied by squatters or informal settlements, and – at the other end of the wealth spectrum – by those seeking environmental amenity through coastal canal estates, and riverside and bush locations, areas that are often at greater risk from floods and fires.

The growth of urbanization

Much of the hazards literature argues that large contemporary cities – 'megacities' – are incubators for disasters because of the concentration of people and activities in a confined space and the generation of new hazards (Mitchell, 1999; Pelling, 2003). However, although less so in poorer countries, this situation can be balanced by the fact that cities contain massive resources to cope with hazards. In addition, the growth of cities may also be an adaptation against other forms of hazard, including lawlessness and climatic hazards such as drought. The overall situation is unclear; but cities are growing very rapidly and now contain about half of humanity. Unfortunately, this is often closely associated with environmental degradation, such as the removal of the natural protection against storms and flooding provided by mangroves, wetlands and sand dunes.

Economic and social factors, and rapid change

In wealthy areas, increasing wealth and exposure of wealth in existing hazardous locations is a primary driver of escalating disaster losses. The UK's study of future flood losses (Foresight, 2004) highlights this issue. In these circumstances, high losses largely offset by insurance are not by themselves indicators of low resilience.

In contrast, economic globalization, chronic corruption, aspects of economic 'structural adjustment programmes' and the changes accompanying the collapse of communism and other forms of highly centralized government (such as in Eastern Europe) are examples of social factors that often undermine people's capacity to cope with hazards. Many countries have serious problems of corruption and weak institutions. These factors inhibit development and people's ability to improve their lives and prospects, undermining and even reversing progress on key contributors to resilience, such as healthcare, political representation, mobility and livelihood security, and the capacity of government to plan for, and respond to, crises.

Economic globalization is seen as an unqualified good by almost all political leaders in the industrialized world. The essence of the argument is that through free trade, the whole world will become more prosperous. However, many poorer countries and those working with poorer sections of society worldwide might disagree. Focusing on distributional issues, they cite as evidence the growing gulf between nations, and between rich and poorer people within countries (e.g. Stiglitz, 2002), with the accompanying implication that their vulnerability is increasing and their ability to cope with emergencies is declining.

Dispossession by war or civil strife

Refugees and those driven into marginal areas are often the most dramatic examples of people vulnerable to the negative effects of natural events, cut off from coping mechanisms and support networks. About half of the world's countries are directly linked to uprooted populations, with people being forced to flee in some 60 countries (US Committee for Refugees, 2000). Where warfare is involved, these areas are also characterized by an exodus of trained people and an absence of inward investment. Reasons for the increase in vulnerability associated with warfare include destruction or abandonment of infrastructure (transport, communications, health and education) and shelter; redirection of resources from social to military purposes; collapse of trade and commerce; abandonment of subsistence farmlands; and lawlessness and disruption of social networks (Levy and Sidel, 2000). The proliferation of weapons and minefields, the absence of basic health and education, and the collapse of livelihoods can ensure that the effects of war on vulnerability to disasters are long lasting.

Evolution of emergency management: From 'acts of God' to socially constructed disasters

The above list of causal factors shows the overriding importance of human factors – social, economic and political – in generating vulnerability to disaster and exacerbating the impacts of natural phenomena. By comparison, natural phenomena, over which we have little or no control, often make relatively modest contributions to disaster vulnerability. This statement must be qualified for those whose livelihoods depend entirely on climate, and for exceptionally severe events such as the Asian tsunami, which may have very serious impacts at the local level, especially in poor countries and poor regions of otherwise wealthy countries.

Overall, though, thinking has shifted in emergency management from being dominated by a passive, accepting approach – disasters as 'acts of God' – with the resulting attitude that little can be done, to a more proactive approach that accepts the role of humans in creating the conditions for disasters. This opens the way for the development of institutions, policy and practice aimed at reducing vulnerability and enhancing resilience. Recognizing the importance of human agency, however, may also encourage attribution of blame, whether deservedly or not, so the shift is by no means entirely positive.

Modern emergency management involves many players with distinctive backgrounds and reasons for involvement. In some countries, these organizations have their origins in the 'civil defence' or 'home guard' units developed during World War II. Working with the career uniformed services and established welfare groups, such as the Red Cross and the Salvation Army, they supported the home front. After the war, it was not long before there was another threat that had a military aspect – the Cold War and the possibility of nuclear attack – creating the imperative for maintaining civil defence capacities. Although the precise evolution varied by jurisdiction, such war-related organizations found themselves increasingly busy with more 'everyday' emergencies and crises arising from natural agents and from transport and technological failures: events that affected and concerned far more people than hypothetical risks of war. During the 1970s, most civil defence organizations in Western countries formally shifted focus in terms of their corporate image to an emergency management, rather than war-related, emphasis. Civil defence was not about risk management as such – it did not attempt to reduce threat of war, but rather sought to protect the state and, to a lesser extent, the people.

In thinking about emergency management organizations, we need to be aware that the key groups include many dedicated more to recovery and support than the actual task of immediate response. This is especially the case in the non-governmental and government welfare sector. The culture, interest and background of these groups are quite different from emergency management organizations and are largely complementary to them.

We are not critical of a strong response focus – that is what society, media and politicians want when a crisis erupts. It saves lives and property and is indispensable and utterly admirable. Rather, we advocate a greater *additional* emphasis on strategic thinking and policy, while maintaining a high level of response capability. Recent shifts in thinking in emergency management are in keeping with our position, and are summarized in Table 1.2. We argue for an intensification of these trends.

Recent trends in disaster and emergency research and management reflect a range of interests, some of them common to other public policy areas, such as sustainable development:

- seeking to put emergency management into the policy mainstream and away from a marginal activity by reframing problems;
- seeking to deal with causes rather than symptoms, emphasizing the need for learning and greater efforts in strategic policy development;
- the need for appropriate institutional structures to deliver long-term solutions;
- sharing ownership of the problem with those at risk and working to reduce vulnerability.

Generally, we can say that among many in the social and policy sciences, adaptation to hazards and sustainable development are now seen as interlocking aims (Mileti, 1999). The World Summit on Sustainable Development (WSSD), the ten year follow-on to the first United Nations Conference on Environment and Development (UNCED) of 1992, was held in 2002 in Johannesburg. The summit made disaster reduction one of its central themes. To be very vulnerable is not sustainable – economically, environmentally or socially.

In summary, today emergency management is largely about being resilient in the

Table 1.2 *Trends in emergency management*

From	To
Framing the fundamental issue:	
Hazards as 'other' – acts of God	Hazards are generated by humans
Event driven	Situational and less visible creeping hazards included
Policy context:	
Lack of visibility and profile	Legal liability
	Rising expectations and critical scrutiny
	Impacts of counter-terrorism and security
Problem ownership and framing:	
Acceptance/individual decision-making	Community vulnerability and
Local	sustainability
Choice	Local–global
	Institutional constraints
Style:	
Secret	Open
Paramilitary	Dominantly civilian
Uncertainty ignored or quantified	Uncertainty is acknowledged
Policy emphasis:	
Accept or reduce loss	Manage vulnerability or increase
Focus on the hazard and event	resilience
Solutions as separate	Focus on community safety and consequences
	Solutions found in organization of society and the development process

Source: Drawing on Handmer (2003b)

face of uncertainty. This involves a shift – easier in concept than in practice – from treating symptoms to dealing with causes. In turn, this is closely linked with the emphasis on addressing vulnerability through building capacity and resilience in communities at risk. In some cases, a fundamental shift in thinking has occurred so that causes are redefined or reframed, particularly to recognize human agency and structures rather than fate, and to clarify what we are trying to achieve. Once human agency is recognized, the problem becomes more amenable to policy intervention.

Redefining the problem and objectives can be a powerful mechanism of change (explored further in Chapter 5). For example, Merseyside fire service in the UK examined the pattern of urban fires, including arson, and identified poverty as the critical underlying factor (McGurk, 2005). The fire service cannot do much about poverty directly, but has changed its approach radically by incorporating this information. At a general level, for commercial enterprises, the first need is usually to minimize disruption so that trade can continue, rather than simply preventing physical damage; and for many communities, protection of the livelihood base is usually the first priority, rather than reconstructing buildings. The institutional setting needs to be amenable to this type of strategic and creative thinking, where underlying causes are targeted.

Examples can inform better ways of constructing disasters as problems, and identifying what comes before and after a disaster event, thus informing strategic approaches. We now turn to a series of vignettes to expose and illustrate the themes that the rest of the book will pursue.

Illustrative vignettes

The following brief case studies illustrate both success and failure in terms of the broad policy and institutional response of vertical or horizontal coordination, accountability, participation, evaluation and information on risks, and short-term decision imperatives, among other issues. Boxes 1.1 to 1.9 identify themes and challenges that are addressed in later chapters. Table 1.3 matches the 'vignette' cases studies and the themes that the book focuses on and is organized around. The vignettes deliberately describe disasters of a massive scale, well known to the world, as well as others of smaller extent and impact, but which nonetheless illustrate generic issues. We can learn from experiences both large and small, and certainly must respond to both.

Table 1.3 *The book's themes and illustrative case studies*

Book themes				
Long, complex antecedents	Hurricane Katrina	London	The Netherlands	Goma
Disasters and development impacts	Asian tsunami	Mozambique	Goma	
Owning the problem/ accountability	Hurricane Katrina	Longford	London	
Problem framing	Asian tsunami	Goma	Nyngan	The Netherlands
Responding and implementing: policy choice	Asian tsunami	Goma	The Netherlands	
Learning from experience	Nyngan	The Netherlands	Australian wildfire	
Institutional settings	Hurricane Katrina	Longford	Mozambique	

Box 1.1 *Hurricane Katrina, New Orleans, US*

Much of the city of New Orleans – a city of over 1 million inhabitants – lies below sea level, and much of the surrounding land of the Mississippi delta has been eroding away for decades. Within days of warning, Hurricane Katrina headed towards New Orleans in August 2005, creating a storm surge that forced itself into the lakes and canals surrounding and bisecting the city, and breached and/or overtopped levees protecting the city. The majority of those at risk evacuated in some chaos as a normally short drive took most of the day. However, over 100,000 people (including many tourists) did not evacuate, either lacking the means to do so or deciding to stay.

Neither the hurricane striking the city, nor the inability of over 100,000 people to evacuate should have been a surprise. The whole event, generally and in detail, was well predicted and thoroughly rehearsed. A report in *Nature* soon after the event observed that 'The similarities between Katrina and the Hurricane Pam simulation (used for training by emergency management agencies at the various levels of government) are eerie' (Reichhardt et al, 2005).

However, while the event was expected, the outcomes were surprising. The predictions, scenarios and rehearsals did not deal with the paralysis of local and state government that occurred; the collapse of essential services (which appears to have continued to worsen as organizations ran into financial problems); the sense that law and order had broken down; the abandonment of many of the more vulnerable people; the thousands of children separated from their parents; and the seeming inability of the federal government to come to terms with the scope and nature of the disaster.

It was assumed, and in many cases asserted, that planning and preparations were thorough and would be effective. It was well known from the various disaster planning scenarios that a car-based evacuation would leave some 100,000 stranded. This occurred and those stranded were also those who had played the most limited role in previous emergency planning – marginalized or poor residents and tourists. The stranded were eventually evacuated to points scattered throughout the US. The media and state and local officials gave full ownership of the resulting problems to the US federal government and particularly to the Federal Emergency Management Agency (FEMA) and its parent agency, the Department of Homeland Security (DHS). Local and state officials avoided responsibility, and no one seemed interested in owning the problem or even in gaining political capital from dealing with it (Handmer, 2006):

> Katrina exposed serious problems in our response capability at all levels of government, and to the extent that the federal government didn't fully do its job, I take responsibility. (President Bush, BBC, 13 September 2005)

The planning had been thorough in many respects, but failed to include many key players, and this was reflected in the response that was slow to take advantage of private-sector and major NGO capacity. This form of exclusion from emergency policy and planning is by no means confined to Hurricane Katrina. This exposes the challenge of intergovernmental and cross-sectoral coordination (see Chapters 2 and 8).

The government reports into the Katrina and New Orleans disaster are clear: there was a failure of leadership at all levels. This may seem rather harsh. Why should one or two people carry the blame for the failure of very large organizations in a major crisis? There was a failure to clarify ownership of the almost infinite number of issues and problems by all those involved, and there were institutional failures not only within the key organizations responsible for disaster response and recovery, but also with inter-organizational coordination. Strategic failures in planning and thinking are linked to these issues and are also seen in the inability to deal with an event that is large in space and time – and with an apparent failure to take account of the local political and socio-economic context, even though it was very well known and documented. The biggest failure may be emerging in the apparent lack of direction about the future of New Orleans and the regional economy.

There is now argument over the 'real' extent of the crisis. However, there is little argument over the absence of clear decisions and recovery direction, even two years on. Much of the aid and livelihood support had conditions attached that made its utility limited or were strictly time limited. The evidence is mounting that there was limited strategic planning before the event, and that officials have struggled to find any since. Another view is that there was substantial strategic and response planning, but that it was poorly connected to the vulnerabilities of people at risk, as well as to the institutional and geophysical realities.

Box 1.2 *Longford gas explosion, Victoria, Australia*

An explosion and fire on 25 September 1998 halted gas production at Esso's Longford plant in the Australian state of Victoria. Two employees were killed and eight others injured. Supplies of natural gas to domestic and industrial users were halted for over two weeks. The Longford plant was the primary source of Victoria's gas, and only very small amounts of gas were available to Victorians during the crisis through an emergency supply from a pipeline link with the neighbouring state of New South Wales and a small gas field in Victoria. Victorians had also experienced a cut in their supplies from Longford following an incident at the plant earlier the same year.

Much industry depends on gas supplies, as do hospitals and schools, and there were some 200 individuals who used gas-powered life-support systems. The state faced an energy crisis that could easily become a political and economic crisis, in addition to the human impact (Hopkins, 2000).

The State Premier, emergency services and industry worked to make the problem everyone's problem. The Premier made it clear that everyone in the state would be sharing the burden, and that working together to overcome the difficulties posed was the only way of ensuring that the state's industries, employment and essential services would be maintained and that no group would prosper at the expense of others. The small amount of gas available went to essential services and some industries. The emergency services, including the Department of Human Services, which has charge of disaster recovery coordination, worked to identify and support the most vulnerable and worst affected. It had been assumed that the elderly would be in this group; but that was not the case.

To prevent a complete run-down of reserves, supplies of gas were prioritized to essential services only, such as hospitals. About 1.3 million households and 89,000 businesses were affected by the disaster and export earnings alone were cut by over AU$200 million. Stand downs and production losses for affected Victorian and interstate businesses and factories were initially estimated by the Victorian Employer's Chamber of Commerce and Industry to cost billions of dollars, a figure later revised to AU$1.3 billion, as reported by the *Financial Review* on 27 April 1999.

On 2 October 1998, a AU$100 million federal government assistance package was announced for Victorians affected by gas shortages. The government lost about AU$300 million in tax revenue. The disaster triggered the largest class action in the country's history with 10,000 claimants. However, this and other similar legal actions were later dismissed by the courts. The final restoration of gas supply to all consumers took place by 14 October 1998.

The Premier of Victoria re-commissioned the Longford Gas Plant on 13 March 2002. The plant was rebuilt at a cost of AU$500 million and incorporated new safety measures and staffing increases. Esso also announced that it would invest a further AU$100 million in the development and expansion of the Longford plant over the next two years (Premier of Victoria, Australia, News Archive, 13 March 2002).

The Victorian government has established gas supply redundancies, in part by including other suppliers, and has acted on the recommendations of the Longford Royal Commission, including the implementation of a rigorous safety regime for hazardous sites. Emergency management agencies, especially the Department of Human Services, which shouldered much of the work, has altered its procedures and established mechanisms to manage large disasters of this kind (Hopkins, 2000).

This is not to suggest that the crisis was handled perfectly, but that the various levels of government and sectors in Victoria worked well together to handle a major infrastructure failure, and later to increase the resiliency of the system. Information for Longford came primarily from the EMATrack database, maintained by Emergency Management Australia.

Box 1.3 *The South Asian tsunami*

The 26 December 2004 tsunami swept 8000km across the Indian Ocean in a matter of hours, inundating coastal areas of Indonesia, Thailand, India, Sri Lanka, the Maldives, Somalia and Malaysia, among others, resulting in some 300,000 deaths and enormous physical damage in various locations. The tsunami was generated by a very powerful undersea earthquake just offshore from the Indonesian province of Aceh. There were no warnings, although some people were saved by informal alerts.

The resilience of many coastal areas – in terms of local livelihoods – depends upon income through tourism. Should the area suffer some major shock, the longer-term effect will be related to the ability of the area to recover from this impact. The tsunami of 2004 devastated many tourism areas, including some in southern Thailand. Resorts were destroyed, many local people and international tourists were killed, and the areas suffered something approaching the worst possible publicity as countless people searched for their missing friends and relatives against a backdrop of devastation.

Recovery and the longer-term survival and prosperity of the affected areas depend, as they frequently do following disaster, upon the vitality of the local economy. This means that the flows of money into and within an area affected by disaster needs to reach those affected. However, increasingly this is framed within the context of a globalized economy, and the restoration of high-profile assets – referred to as 'thing theory' in the *2001 World Disasters Report* – may not be well connected to the livelihoods of local people (IFRC, 2001).

Most of the local survivors lost their employment and normal livelihoods. Some governments, such as Australia, urged their citizens to leave the area immediately after the tsunami and to return home – thereby depriving the areas of desperately needed foreign exchange and employment. In one sense, this highlights that disaster planning and thinking may need to be concerned with economies and livelihoods in other countries.

Although the approach of supporting local commerce, where possible, may seem obvious, it is not universally accepted among economists (IFRC, 2001). The Red Cross uses the analogy of a leaking bucket, where 'plugging the leaks ensures that post-disaster resources re-circulate within the local economy, rather than leaking out of it' (IFRC, 2001). Although this idea is based more on recovery in poorer economies, the approach can also be applied in developed nations, especially in rural communities where aid funds are less likely to re-circulate.

For most of the world and some sectors within rich countries, understanding the informal economy is the key to understanding people's livelihoods and the necessary emphasis on survival, rather than wealth or profit accumulation. It is often celebrated by sociologists as showing people's resilience in the face of economic systems that do not offer anything to them. Others, such as the World Bank, see the informal sector (known less favourably as the 'black economy') as something to be eliminated, arguing that it is primarily a tax dodge and connected with over-regulation (see Handmer and Choong, 2006).

Box 1.4 *Wildfire evacuation in Australia*

Learning from experience, with a major impact on policy, can occur incrementally as a result of a number of events and subsequent analysis, rather than simply arising from a single event or as a result of research and a bureaucratic process of adoption and change. The adoption of the wildfire evacuation policy in Australia provides an example.

In parts of Australia, there has been an emphasis on avoiding last minute evacuations, now formalized in a position on community safety and evacuation during bushfires summed up by the catch phrase: 'Houses protect people and people protect houses.' The basic message of the Australasian Fire Authorities Council (AFAC) is that where adequate fire protection measures have been implemented, able-bodied people should be encouraged to stay with their homes in the event of wildfire. This position moves away from the evacuation doctrine that has prevailed among emergency services during recent decades towards greater community self-reliance. It is referred to as the 'Prepare, stay and defend or leave early' policy, and it is now widely endorsed by Australian wildfire-fighting agencies.

In the Stay or Go approach, 'staying' means preparing, staying and actively defending the property as the fire front passes, and from ember attack before and after the front. 'Going' means making a decision not to defend the property and leaving well before the fire front arrives. Findings on how houses burn down and what happens to people when they adopt different behaviour in the face of a fire, demonstrating significantly higher survival of houses when defended, were used to develop the approach.

The first post-war iconic Australian urban interface fire occurred in Hobart, Tasmania, on 7 February 1967. It resulted in 62 deaths and the loss of 1300 homes, and led to investigations of house and personal survivals. Findings by Alan McArthur and Phil Cheney of the Commonwealth Scientific and Industrial Research Organization's (CSIRO's) Forest Research Institute found that:

> Most of the people who died in their homes or within a short distance thereof were either very old and infirm, or suffered from some physical disability. In the case of about half of the people who died whilst escaping from their homes, such homes did not catch fire. In a few cases it may be said that if they had stayed inside they would have had a reasonable chance of survival. (McArthur and Cheney, 1967)

The Ash Wednesday fires of February 1983 destroyed about 2300 buildings and resulted in 83 deaths in the states of Victoria and South Australia. The clearest lesson in the studies following the fires was that late evacuation is dangerous: twice as many deaths occurred in vehicles or in the open than inside houses. Research also showed that the single major determinant of house survival was the presence of able-bodied people. People would extinguish the small ember fires that normally grow to destroy houses, an insight gained during the 1940s.

Analysis of the Australian evidence in support of the policy and its gradual adoption shows a somewhat hesitant process, affected by various institutional and political priorities, such as legal liability, or the desire for clear empirical evidence. Nevertheless, a series of major wildfire disasters, empirical investigation combined with legal inquiries, a desire by senior fire managers to ensure that wildfire policy and practice are based on defensible evidence, and the recent creation of national forums where strategic policy issues can be discussed have seen the approach become national policy. While implementation challenges remain, shared understanding of a fundamental principle has emerged.

This approach also highlights a possible weakness with the international research literature on evacuation. The published material almost invariably frames the evacuation research question in terms of how to get people to leave. There is very little on alternatives and few attempts to frame the problem differently in terms of minimizing risk or loss.

Source: adapted from Handmer and Tibbits (2005)

Box 1.5 *Floods at Nyngan, New South Wales, Australia*

Flood warning systems seem to be characterized by failure; yet, increasingly, our acceptance of risk relies on effective warnings to protect us from the inevitable remaining or residual risk.

In April 1990, the three mainland states of eastern Australia experienced severe flooding. Two country towns (Charleville, with 3200 people, and Nyngan, with 2500 people, in the states of Queensland and New South Wales, respectively) had to be completely evacuated and there were substantial evacuations from small urban centres in the Gippsland area of the state of Victoria, as well. Nyngan, in particular, was a major media and political event, and an exemplary case study of a community repeatedly affected by floods and reliant on ever higher levees as protection (Newell and Wasson, 2002). In 1990, virtually the whole community was involved in placing over 200,000 sandbags to heighten the existing levee that created a dry 'island' on the vast flooded western plains. This environment comprises a very low relief, with meandering, braided streams and the slow exit of floodwaters. Eventually, the augmented levee was overpowered, the town was flooded and the population was evacuated by helicopter – the problem had shifted from protection to escape. The extensive and damaging flooding in the three states put warnings and emergency management under intense public scrutiny.

As a result of the inadequacies in warning system performance, a national workshop on flood warnings was convened by the national coordination agency, Emergency Management Australia, in late 1991, with 50 participants from government (the state and territory Flood Warning Consultative Committees) and non-governmental (media and research) organizations involved in various aspects of the warning task, from flood detection and prediction through to the delivery of warning messages. This workshop ended with a consensus calling for the production of a national guide to good practice in the field of flood warning (EMA, 1999). The guide was published in 1995 and revised in 1999. Great efforts were made to include as many agencies and key individuals as possible in the process of development, and the guide was endorsed by most Australian flood warning-related agencies. However, actual implementation on the ground has been slow in most jurisdictions.

Box 1.6 *Mozambique floods of 2000*

Heavy continuous rainfall across Southern Africa induced flooding on 9 February 2000, and southern Mozambique bore the brunt of the deluge. People started fleeing the capital Maputo as main roads and electricity were cut between the capital and Beira, the second most-populated city. Over 70 people were reported to have died by 11 February as the Limpopo River burst its banks, causing severe flood damage to the Limpopo Valley to the north of Maputo.

Tropical Cyclone Eline hit the coast near Beira, with winds measuring up to 260 kilometres per hour on 22 February 2000. Considered one of the worst floods in living memory, getting relief supplies to affected areas, particularly clean drinking water, was a priority, with relief dependency an ongoing concern during the initial reconnaissance efforts. There was confusion over which aid agency would do what as relief supplies hit the ground. The United Nations and Mozambique government oversaw the entire operation, conducting daily meetings with all aid agencies involved. The cost of rebuilding would add to an already burgeoning external debt that is close to US$8.3 billion, bearing interest of up to US$1.4 million per week. With little ability to return to pre-disaster economic growth levels, the question of debt always surfaces after disaster in developing countries.

The media became a circus, with what was described on the BBC as a 'clash between the face of modern media and global communications and the people of a very remote, very poor, rural lifestyle'. However, the truth is that without the media presence, few in the world would have known about the enormity of this disaster. Like most disasters, there are stories of triumph of the human spirit: in this case, of the communities and their ability to cope despite the damage.

The flood directly and indirectly killed approximately 800 people and affected about 1.5 million more, approximately 12 per cent of the nation's population. Many small farm households lost their livelihoods to damage and many livestock were lost. Nine-tenths of the country's irrigation infrastructure was destroyed, along with industrial urban areas and communications and road infrastructure. The economic cost of relief in itself was very modest at: US$5.9 million for health, US$3.6 million for relief kits, US$3 million for fuel and running costs, and US$6.4 million to rebuild some infrastructure to move relief goods into the country. It is estimated that it will take around ten years to fully recover and rebuild.

Box 1.7 *Flooding in The Netherlands, 1993 and 1995*

Living under the threat of catastrophic flooding is part of the Dutch national ethos, and flood risk is a policy field with a high profile. About half of The Netherlands is protected from flooding by dikes, with about half the population at risk. The risk is mostly from the sea; but a significant risk comes from the Rhine and Meuse (Maas) rivers that flow into The Netherlands, bringing water from other countries. Since 1978, the level of flood protection has been set in legislation at the 1:1250 flood (or 1250-year flood) for riverine flooding. In the upstream area of the Meuse, the population at risk is in the floodplain, parts of which are protected by levees; but downstream and along the Rhine, the people live in polders (areas protected by ring dikes) that can be flooded rapidly with potential for heavy loss of life (van der Grijp and Olsthoorn, 2000).

Responsibilities for disaster planning, management and response are set out in 1985 legislation. Disaster planning is required. At the local level, 572 mayors are in charge of the disaster response organizations, while local fire chiefs have the primary local operational responsibility. Sixty-five water boards are responsible for water-related issues, including dike security. Although warnings are the responsibility of the national water ministry, failure to respect local decision-making authorities can lead to conflict and to mayors overturning provincial decisions to evacuate.

Warnings have traditionally given highest priority to those responsible for dyke protection. This is complicated by the fact that some dikes are centuries old, and lack of knowledge about their construction means that predicting failure is problematic. Post-flood compensation has been provided by government on a generous, if *ad hoc*, basis. Since 1998, this has been formalized by legislation. Flood insurance is not available.

The 1993 flood on the Meuse in the south of The Netherlands occurred just before Christmas as a result of heavy rain in northern France and Belgium. Its ferocity caught emergency services and residents by surprise, and some 10,000 were evacuated. The situation was exacerbated by the absence of communication between the Dutch, Belgian and French authorities, at first, and by the relatively weak state of emergency preparedness.

In 1995, rain in the same areas, in addition to snowmelt were responsible for more serious floods, with over 13,000 houses inundated along the Meuse. Once the authorities responsible for the safety of the dikes protecting the polders along the Rhine announced that they could no longer guarantee their safety, mass evacuation was inevitable. The Mayor of Nijmegen took the lead. There had been considerable learning following the flooding in 1993, and the area had prepared a detailed flood emergency plan, which greatly improved communication and coordination between the various official players, where before there had been little or none. Generally, the authorities were much more proactive in their response. One problem concerned conflict over appropriate warning lead time; but this was settled through 'unofficial' forecasts to emergency managers.

In all, some 250,000 were evacuated in The Netherlands, along with very large numbers of farm animals. It proved to be a largely precautionary measure as the dykes held and the areas flooded along the Meuse were those without full protection. Nevertheless, post-emergency surveys show that nearly all (88 per cent) thought that the evacuation was appropriate (van Duin et al, 1995). To help ensure compliance, the government promised to compensate evacuees for any losses incurred. Investigators suggest that as the initial evacuations (of 60,000 people) in high-risk areas around Nijmegen were successful, it became easier to evacuate other areas. People were very cooperative and those without transportation were largely helped by individuals whom they knew; very few (3 per cent) needed the special buses provided. Local media supported the emergency services, providing information to their audiences.

Box 1.8 *Refugees and a volcano in Goma, Democratic Republic of Congo*

The case of Goma in the Democratic Republic of Congo, and eruption of Mount Nyirangongo, throws light on the complex implications of natural hazards in a society marred by three-and-a-half years of civil war and grappling with serious development issues. The rich volcanic soils and tropical highlands give life to livestock and farming, despite growing migration to urban centres. In January 2002, the city of Goma, on the border with Rwanda, was divided by a wall of black lava that spewed from the volcano into the heart of the city.

Demographically, there is a disproportionately large percentage of young people, many of whom are migrating into regional centres such as Kivu on the Rwanda border. The cross-border Congo–Nile Ridge has become a melting pot for regional instability since 1994, when tens of thousands of Hutu refugees crossed the border. Goma quickly became a rebel city, where Rwandan refugees began re-banding, planning and carrying out cross-border attacks. With the ethnic conflict initiated by the influx of refugees from conflict-ridden Rwanda, the Congo – with the feared regime of Mobuto Sese Seko – caught between warring Hutu and Tutsi rebels and a new leader, Laurant Kibila, experienced developing conflict as Rwanda and Uganda rose up against Kibila, and Zimbabwe, Angola and Namibia backed him as a leader. The situation is far from being a simple volcanic eruption.

On the contrary, this risk context envelops the dimensions of a complex humanitarian conflict; a stagnating formal economy; an unstable political situation both in the country and bordering areas; approximately 95 per cent human displacement from the volcano alone; a refugee crisis; food and water shortage; risk of disease spread through poor sanitation; and damaged infrastructure and transportation routes. Further complicating the matter, there is no clear knowledge of the refugee population that has moved across the border to Rwanda, which makes reaching the survivors for short-term survival needs and long-term resettlement even more difficult. It is said that the numbers reported to have crossed the border are grossly overestimated, and people have been reported as saying: 'They would rather die in their homesteads than in a foreign land where they are not welcome' (Oxfam, 2002).

Standard relief problems are being played out, such as the need to distribute water, shelter and food; but one problem is to avoid creating ongoing dependency among the refugee population, who are now entangled with the residents of many areas, such as Sake, where people have been experiencing severe malnutrition even before the hazard struck.

The case of the Congo reflects the complexities that a natural hazard can place on a country or region when there are existing and/or brewing conflicts. This seems to be a human-induced insecurity and risk situation, catalysed by a natural phenomenon, uncovering a host of layers that add to peoples' livelihood insecurity.

Source: adapted from OECD (2003) and BBC (http://news.bbc.co.uk/1/hi/world/africa/1767789.stm)

Box 1.9 *London smog: Long antecedent, slow response*

The great London smog of 1952 lasted for five days from 5 to 9 December. It resulted in at least 4000 deaths, although retrospective estimates put the death toll as high as 12,000 (Bell and Davis, 2001; Davis, 2002). There were some 100,000 cases of illness directly attributable to the smog, and the city came to a near standstill. It is an example of a disaster slowly building over centuries. The response too was slow and, in a negative sense, strategic as health was traded against money and other priorities.

As long ago as the 13th century, air pollution was recognized as a public health problem in British cities, and the burning of coal was identified as the principal source. Elevated death tolls were attributed to air pollution throughout the 19th century. Although the fog was natural, it trapped sulphur dioxide from coal fires and other industrial toxins. A study by Sir Napier Shaw in 1900 confirmed this phenomenon. A number of studies identified that smoke-laden fogs resulted in many deaths; for example, there was little argument that smog killed 1000 Glaswegians in 1909. The worst affected part of London was usually the working class East End, where the density of factories and domestic dwellings was very high and the low-lying topography trapped the smog (Brimblecombe, 1987).

In 1952, it was unusually cold and the fires were burning more coal than usual; the resulting gases, along with industrial effluent, were trapped by an inversion. Visibility in parts of London dropped to near zero, and nurses report having had trouble seeing to the end of hospital wards. People were dying outside as there was no room for them in hospitals. The first indicator of mass deaths was a shortage of coffins and flowers.

The disaster was well documented, and the post-war political and social context was quite different from before the war. For example, Victorian-era governments had been careful not to interfere with what people could do in their own homes. Clean air legislation was passed in the form of the 1954 City of London (Various Powers) Act and the 1956 and 1968 Clean Air Acts. These acts restricted emissions of black smoke and decreed that residents of urban areas and operators of factories must convert to smokeless fuels.

As a result, the episode is often used as an example of an event triggering appropriate response. However, it may be a better example of the opposite. Governments suspected that smog caused mass deaths for centuries (there was a short-lived attempt to ban coal fires in 1273), and for at least one century the cause–effect link was known. Following the 1952 smog, the government of the day resisted passing legislation for as long as it could, blaming an influenza epidemic for many of the deaths (now discredited; see Bell and Davis, 2001) and trying to link later episodes to smoking. When the legislation was passed, there was a period of many years given for conversions, and it emphasized 'best practicable means', rather than specifying ambient conditions. For industry, the result was tall chimneys. It was only gradually enforced following other mass death episodes – for example, in 1957 and in 1962, when about 800 Londoners died as a result of smog. Further improvements have come gradually, in part as a result of the decline of polluting industry within London, and in part driven by the European Commission. The episode and its associated public and professional debates and government action make it a landmark in the environmental health movement.

Source: adapted from Brimblecombe (1987); Bell and Davis (2001); Davis (2002); further information was gleaned from the BBC and UK Met Office websites (http://news.bbc.co.uk/2/hi/health/2545747.stm; www.metoffice. com/education/secondary/students/smog.html)

Key challenges

These vignettes of disasters and the discussion of how they were understood and handled illustrate important themes, including those proposed in Table 1.3. We can iterate these themes now, all of which will be explored further in later chapters, and which are located largely in the second column of Table 1.2: the future of disaster and emergency management, rather than its past and present.

The report by the US National Science and Technology Council (2005), *Grand Challenges for Disaster Reduction*, argues that 'Communities must break the cycle of destruction and recovery by enhancing their disaster resilience.' It advocates information, behaviour change and the application of new technologies. The mission of the UN's International Strategy for Disaster Reduction (ISDR) promotes a similar mission, although without a technology emphasis: 'The ISDR aims to build disaster-resilient communities by promoting increased awareness of the importance of disaster reduction as an integral part of sustainable development' (UN–ISDR, 1999).

These and many other statements by political and scientific leaders – often made in the immediate aftermath of a catastrophe – highlight that, for many, disaster reduction will result from the application of technology, as well as the need for increased community awareness as a prelude for improvement. These are important parts of a disaster reduction programme but, like other aspects of resilience, are frequently hindered by the absence of a strategic policy framework to support improved prevention, preparedness, response and recovery. We attempt to address the latter need. In doing so, important themes or challenges are as follows:

- Disasters and emergencies are a *whole-of-society problem*, and thus also a whole-of-government problem, and are especially a joint concern of responsible government and potentially affected communities. Thus, the ownership of the problem, and participation in response, are wider than often assumed in a traditional preparedness-response approach. Wider ownership of the problem necessitates different policy processes and policy responses, based on different relationships, information and sources of authority. Ownership of, and participation in managing, the problem requires recognition of community vulnerability and resilience, including non-tangible aspects such as spiritual values, non-economic attachment to place, cultural assets and continuity, and the informal economy.
- The importance of initial *problem framing*, including clear identification of proximate versus underlying causes. Put simply, the problem can be construed as: people are at risk of flooding, and levees and evacuation assistance are needed; or disadvantaged groups (or rich individuals with political influence) are living in flood-prone areas, and while levees and assistance should be provided, livelihoods issues, lack of alternative housing and planning laws should be considered. Community *vulnerability and resilience* become primary concerns, in local economic and asset terms, as well as aspects such as cultural identity, lay knowledge, health, local institutions, etc.
- The inevitability of *residual risk and uncertainty*. No matter what the quantity and quality of knowledge or the sophistication of policy and management, unexpected events, human behaviours and complex phenomena will place people and places at risk and confound our presumed understanding. Explicit admission of residual uncertainty in the natural and built environment, government institutions and local vulnerabilities reinforces the need for contingency planning, positive redundancies and safety margins, a flexible and adaptive response capacity, and better shared understanding of the circumstances of vulnerability.
- *Redundancy.* In the past, including some redundancy in our systems may be sound practice not simply for emergency management, but also for enterprises operating in the face of uncertainty and with much at stake. Nevertheless, this is seen as inefficient and suboptimal in a commercial world dedicated to being productive. The issue for emergency managers is that a small failure in

any part of such 'optimized' systems is likely to amplify through the rest of the system. Charles Perrow (1984) calls these highly sensitive arrangements tightly coupled systems. In rich countries, this is well demonstrated by just-in-time food and energy distribution systems that may be highly vulnerable to disruption. Conversely, advancing technology means that telecommunication systems may now have built-in redundancy through the parallel use of landlines and mobile phones. Our argument is not for built-in *inefficiency*, but for consideration of the impacts of failure and the use of 'fail-safe' design where appropriate – some of this may come from harnessing informal or community capacity. In this book we apply these ideas to policy and institutions, rather than to the more usual focus on back-up technology and operational capacity.

- *Strategic policy development*. Emergency management has, understandably, been mainly concerned with dealing with the immediacy of crises: it has been good at management, but not at strategy. Efforts at strategic thinking have often been constrained by long-established standard models and approaches. An issue is that many of the constituents of vulnerability and resilience are found in the organization of daily life, and in the culture and priorities of government and corporations – and are not easily addressed by emergency managers. This sets up the challenge of how strategic policy capacity can be created and implemented.
- The art and craft of *policy instrument choice* for disaster management requires development in terms of the range of options considered, the basis for their selection and the inclusiveness of the policy formulation process. In addition, *policy implementation* is often under-attended, particularly in the lull between disaster events, when political and public attention wanders and strategies are starved of resources.
- Long-term *learning and purposeful adaptation* of response strategies could be greatly improved, again particularly across the attention peaks associated with irregular disaster events. This and the other imperatives above emphasize the importance of the *institutional settings* defining the ongoing capacities and strategies in the disasters and emergency field.
- *Multiple aims and values* – reducing the impacts and consequences of disaster is a core aim of emergency management agencies; but this aim is usually interpreted in multiple ways and pursued through locally specific political, administrative and legal institutions, consistent with the priorities of these institutions. Priorities may include commercialization of services; development rather than hazard management; aid intended to buy political influence rather than to assist victims; privileging 'national security' over other needs; avoiding controversy; detailed auditing and real-time record-keeping; and so on. Some aims and values will not be stated explicitly, but are embedded in organizational culture and include priorities that undermine disaster programmes. Legal frameworks may inhibit decision-making as those responsible consider potential legal liabilities. They may also have budget constraints, although the post-disaster impact surge in expenditure may lead to a local economic boom in some circumstances. The administrative aim may be to reduce expenditure, transferring the risk to the individuals involved or to the private sector. Whether these constraints are real or not, they can limit the space for decisions. Some senior emergency managers argue that *perception is reality*. Political

and media priorities for the dramatic and immediate, or an individual's agenda for hero status, can also turn perceptions into reality as far as the emergency manager is concerned and make long-term learning difficult. Explicitly including multiple aims and values in emergency policy and planning is one approach to managing these issues.

Some of these themes and their associated dimensions are addressed within the structure of the book, such as policy instrument choice in Chapter 6. Others, such as community resilience, emerge in a number of chapters. Following the argument that thinking about disasters and emergencies has focused more on management than on policy, Chapter 2 surveys key ideas in policy and institutional studies in terms of their relevance to disasters.

2

The Nature of Policy and Institutions

Policy and institutions are commonplace terms and complex phenomena that pervade our lives. They are at once terms and phenomena that we live with, construct and change, battle against and have opinions about. The policy processes, programmes and instruments, and the institutional systems through which policies emerge, impact on, and are designed to direct, the behaviour of individuals, households, communities, firms, organizations and societies in order to achieve social goals. Policies may be well designed or not, and may succeed or not. If society wishes to better understand, avoid, prepare for or cope with emergencies and disasters, then over the long term, this can only be achieved through effective policy processes operating within suitable institutional settings.

Policy and institutions are the subjects of a massive body of theoretical and practical knowledge, inside individuals' heads, in government organizations and in a wide body of scholarly and professional literature. Individuals, professional and academic societies, public and private organizations, and university departments and programmes focus on policy and institutions. Yet, often such policy knowledge is discounted, and we merely argue using simple opinions about 'policy', rather than engage in constructive discourse based on shared understanding.

This chapter presents a summary discussion on the nature of policy and institutions. This is not a policy text: the aim is to extract from the general public policy literature key ideas of relevance to disasters. Readers are referred to more detailed sources. The chapter first defines core terms and concepts, then summarizes key ideas. It then places policy in the context of the contemporary political environment, and characterizes emergencies and disasters as policy and institutional problems.

Abrupt and unexpected change – including emergencies and disasters – challenge standard policy processes and policy settings and the ways of thinking that underpin these, throw policy processes and institutions into chaos, devastate lives and communities, and even cause governments to fall. Sometimes, the scale of an event makes this inevitable; sometimes policy systems should have been better prepared. While this chapter focuses on traditional public policy, the poor fit between 'policy as usual' and 'emergencies as exceptions' is an underlying theme, and will be further explored in Chapter 3 and later chapters.

Core concepts and terms

'Policy' and 'institutions' are the subjects of this book and are of crucial importance in how societies conceive of, and respond to, emergencies and disasters. The two terms, however, are used by policy practitioners, academic disciplines and in everyday language in divergent ways. In strict theoretical terms, an institution is an underlying rule or pattern within a society; yet, in everyday language, it might be used to refer to a particular organization, physical object or even an individual – for example, a local bank, a building long occupied by the same business and function, or the old man who always occupies the same seat at the bus stop. Particular academic disciplines have strict definitions of what policy means that vary from those of other disciplines. Although complete precision and agreement over terminology are not possible, nor even perhaps desirable, we will propose and use the following set of terms and concepts for consistency:[1]

- *Institutions* are persistent, predictable arrangements, laws, processes or customs serving to structure transactions and relationships in a society. These transactions are political, social, cultural, economic, personal, legal and administrative. Institutions may be informal or formal, legal or customary, and in terms of function may be economic, cultural or informational, highly visible and regulatory, or, alternatively, difficult to discern and relying on tacit understanding and adherence. Institutions allow organized, collective efforts around common concerns, and reduce the need for constant negotiation of expectations and behavioural contracts. Although persistent, institutions constantly evolve and adapt.
- The concept of an *institutional system* conveys the reality that concentrating on single institutions will often limit understanding. Institutions operate within complex, interactive systems comprising multiple institutions, organizations and actors. Describing, analysing or prescribing policy change must take this interdependency into account.
- *Organizations* are manifestations of underlying institutions – specific departments, associations, agencies, etc. In a particular context, an organization may be sufficiently long lived, recognizable and influential to be regarded as an institution; but, generally, organizations can be more quickly dissolved or radically changed than an institution (a government agency manifests institutional traditions of a system of government, and can be renamed, merged or given a revised mandate literally overnight).
- *(Public) policies* are positions taken and communicated by governments in more or less detail – 'avowals of intent' that recognize a problem and state what will be done about it. Policies emerge through complex and variable *policy processes* that include both government and non-government players. Although reflecting the institutions of governance in a jurisdiction, policy processes vary greatly across issues, sectors and over time. The term *policy cycle* is synonymous here with policy process, emphasizing the cyclic and reiterative nature of policy-making. Policy system is a related term, and *policy sub-systems* refer to the fact that, within the broader landscape of public policy in a jurisdiction, somewhat separate sets

of processes and actors exist for specific sectors or issues. In other words, one can delineate the policy sub-system concerned with emergency management, as opposed to public health policy (but also recognize likely overlaps and links).

- Private or community organizations also develop, communicate and seek to implement policies; however, the focus here is on *public policy*, which may nonetheless reflect or even be dictated by the policy positions or proposals of non-government organizations. The crucial difference is that public policies are enabled by the democratic legitimacy and legal authority of government.

- *Policy style* describes the general nature of policy-making in a jurisdiction, government or political system, ranging from legally based, coercive styles dominated by government, to 'corporatist' traditions where policy is negotiated with major interest groups, to a reliance on local communities. Policy styles vary from country to country, and within countries over time as conditions and social values change or as administrations of a different political persuasion win government. A single government or society may also employ different styles according to the nature of issues faced, such as in the case of a rapidly emerging threat.

- *Policy programmes* are specified and substantial manifestations of a policy, comprising elements of implementation, as well as of intent. Beneath this level, for an applied policy, there will be specific and practical projects. For example, a *policy* on community flood preparedness might include a *programme* of community-based flood protection and evacuation plans, and within that programme numerous discrete *projects*, implementing the programme in different locations.

- Public policies are influenced and formulated by multiple *policy actors* as individuals and in organized groups, including politicians, government officials, NGOs, lobbyists and the media. In a democratic system, all voters have some degree of influence; however, surrounding an issue there will be a discernible *policy community*, comprising those who are actively involved in policy discussion. The relative power and influence of members of the policy community varies widely. Within this, a smaller *policy network* will have responsibility for policy formulation and implementation, sharing a reasonably coherent set of beliefs and aspirations.

- Within a policy network or sub-system, there are those termed 'policy- or decision-makers' – this can be an imprecise term. Here, policy- or decision-makers are those with *responsible authority*: the legal competence and mandate within the relevant *jurisdiction* (nation, state or province, local government area, etc.) to make formal policy decisions regarding the matter at hand. The responsible authority may be an individual (e.g. minister or secretary, senior official with *delegated authority* from government, or a court) or an organization (such as a cabinet, statutory body, industry association, firm or community organization). In any significant policy formulation and implementation exercise, more than one responsible authority will likely be involved, making multiple formal decisions on different aspects of the policy response.

- *Policy instruments* are the 'tools' used by governments in partnership with other players to implement policies and achieve policy goals – for example, a regulation, education campaign, tax, intergovernmental agreement or assessment procedure.

- *Management* here refers to actions taken 'on the ground' in implementing a policy instrument and undertaking physical actions. Thus, policy sets the direction, whereas management does things to achieve that direction. Managers and policy-makers may be the same individuals or in the same organization, or may be separate. For example, central government might develop a legally based policy on hazard mapping and preparedness, and a local authority or community-based emergency group may implement this at a local level. *Management regimes* refer to multiple related components through which management actions take place, including regulations, agencies and official monitoring programmes, and funding.

In this book, we will be as consistent as possible with these definitions, acknowledging, however, that the boundaries between both the terms and realities they represent are not always clear, For example, what should strictly be termed an organization may, in a particular context, have the widespread recognition, influence and longevity (and, thus, the ongoing influence on human behaviour) to be thought of as an institution. Likewise, neat divides between the general community, policy community and policy network may not exist. Nonetheless, greater rather than less clarity in terminology assists description, analysis and prescription of 'policy'. The following example, fictional and inevitably somewhat awkward, puts the terms into context:

> In line with the State Emergency Plan (*policy*) and regulations under the Emergencies Act 1999 (legislative *policy instrument*) enabling the State Emergency Management Procedures (related *policy instrument*), the Emergency Services Authority and State Department of Forests (government *organizations*) ordered controlled burning (*management* action) in the state-owned Great Northern Forest. The fire crossed containment lines and damaged assets belonging to adjacent landholders, who took legal action arguing negligence (a legal doctrine within the *institution* of the common law) in the district court (*organization* manifesting that institution). Damages were awarded against the agencies, as represented in the proceedings by their chief executive officers (*responsible authorities*). On advice from the Emergency Services Authority, an independent inquiry, submissions from interested parties (*policy community*) and legal advice (parts of the *policy process*), a government taskforce (*policy network*) developed a new *policy* of negotiated regional fuel-reduction burning plans, reflecting a shift from a top-down regulatory style to an inclusive, cooperative *policy style*.

This indicates the complexity of what lies beneath the terms 'policy' and 'institution', particularly when we recall that the players and context of policy processes vary widely across jurisdictions, time and issues. The stronger focus on emergency *management* than on the policy settings that shape such management – discussed in Chapter 1 – is emphasized in this example as necessarily limited (albeit very important) within the array of equally important concepts and entities that shape societal responses to emergencies and disasters. Making sense of such complexity has challenged policy theorists and practitioners for decades. The next section distils – and sharply summarizes – some key ideas from that body of theory and practice.

Traditions and trends in policy analysis

Notwithstanding deeper roots, the discipline and practice of public policy became prominent following World War II as governments undertook a higher level of intervention in society, in line with the imperatives of reconstruction, rapid growth and change in societies and economies, and the interventionist beliefs of the dominant school of Keynesian economic thought. This represented a new kind and degree of government policy-making and implementation. Social scientists, notably Lasswell (1951, 1971), saw the opportunity and need to bring knowledge and rigour to the enterprise of evolving a new society through active government policy, giving rise to the 'policy sciences'. Over time, there have been many descriptions of that discipline and body of practice, including policy studies, policy analysis, public administration and, most commonly, public policy.

Over the following decades, complicated debates focused on what policy is, who makes policy, and how it can be analysed, made better and evaluated. Rather than trace these ongoing and unresolved debates here, we will simply draw out major issues and themes in public policy. Amidst a massive literature, readers are referred to Finer (1997), Fischer (2003), Howlett and Ramesh (2003), and Peters and Pierre (2003) for detailed, recent and, at times, contrasting texts. Over time, very different views of policy have been put forward. Consider four:

1 The 'rational comprehensive' view sees policy-making as an exact and well-informed problem-solving exercise, where an issue or problem is thoroughly investigated, all possible options are considered, and the optimal policy choice is made. Critics see this as unrealistic, noting that such comprehensiveness is rarely possible in practice, that sufficient information is rarely available and that 'solving' policy problems is a fantasy: in practice, problems are redefined, insufficiently addressed or re-emerge.
2 This was challenged by the 'incremental' view, encapsulated in Lindblom's (1959, 1979) famous phrase: 'the science of muddling through'. He argued that policy change occurs in small steps, taking possible rather than ideal measures, dealing with discrete parts of larger problems. This view is realistic, perhaps; but for many commentators, it is not very strategic or optimal as a way forward.
3 Etzioni (1967) proposed a reasonable half-way compromise – 'mixed scanning' – where an initial and necessarily superficial scoping exercise reduces the policy choices to a manageable few, which can then be analysed and compared in more depth.
4 Depressing but perhaps realistic in some contexts is the 'garbage can model' described by March and Olsen (1979), where ends and means are mixed in a not at all rational rush for answers to emergent problems.

These views represent only four of many theories, and are quite different ways of thinking about policy and about ways of making policy. During recent times, the 'policy cycle' approach has dominated in response to the linear logic of the rational comprehensive model, recognizing the iterative and cyclic nature of policy processes. Reaction against staged 'models' of all kinds is evident, with a counter emphasis on political negotiation and the discursive and contingent nature of policy-making (see below, and Jenkins-Smith and Sabatier, 1994; Healy, 1997; Fischer, 2003).

Despite these recent and well-argued shifts in understanding, it is certainly the case that all four of these approaches are evident in practice, with most, under the right circumstances, being valid. In the case of emergencies and disasters, contexts vary enormously in line with magnitude, uncertainty, onset and vulnerabilities; logically, the nature of policy processes best equipped to cope will vary.

Across all schools of thought, there are a number of persistent themes and questions, and we will now identify these and comment on them very briefly. The aim here is not to resolve such questions, but to recognize them as key themes and uncertainties in thinking about policy so that the later discussion of emergency and disaster policy can take them into account.

Policy analysis: What, why and who?

Public policy as an area of study and practice is multidisciplinary, drawing on insights from political science, public administration, economics, law, sociology and other disciplines. This gives the domain richness and flexibility, but also the characteristic of having multiple sources of perspective and assumptions that underlie methods of policy analysis and policy-making. These underlying beliefs may not always be easily discerned, a point discussed later, but include very different assumptions about how governments work, what motivates human behaviour and the merits of alternative policy styles.

As well as recognizable disciplines, a great deal of policy analysis and design is undertaken by professionals and practitioners who may have an original discipline, but who operate as pragmatic practitioners. In a particular policy sector – such as emergencies and disasters – there will be others whose formal training and expertise are not in a policy-oriented discipline, but who nonetheless are deeply involved in policy debates and, sometimes, policy design. In emergencies and disasters, this may include medical practitioners, information technologists, flood hydrologists and others.

An exercise in policy analysis can have a number of aims and, thus, methods. Fundamental differences include *descriptive* as opposed to *analytical* approaches, and whether *prescription* is attempted. Such differences are explored by Hogwood and Gunn (1984, p29), who separate the categories of policy studies (a neutral pursuit) and policy analysis (a purposeful pursuit), which overlap in the area of evaluation. *Policy studies* are the study of:

- policy content;
- policy process;
- policy outputs;
- evaluation.

Policy analysis involves:

- evaluation;
- information for policy-making;
- process advocacy;
- policy advocacy, with either the analyst as political actor or the political actor as analyst.

There are two lines of distinctions worthy of note here. One allows recognition of the difference between analysis that recommends actual policy options or instruments (*outcomes*) and analysis that evaluates *process*, aimed at improving processes of policy makings. The other is the role and affiliation of the policy analyst – and whether analysts are playing what can be interpreted as a 'political' role driven by value-based concerns, or whether they are taking a more neutral role. While such divisions are at times difficult to make, and an exercise in policy analysis may involve more than one, it is helpful to be clear about such roles and purposes.

Apart from 'formal' academic or professional forms and purposes of engagement with policy, it is clearly the case that, in a policy domain such as emergencies and disasters, all people working in or affected by emergency management do interact with policy in some way, however weakly or indirectly: *policy cannot be avoided* (issues to do with broader public engagement in policy are dealt with in Chapter 4).

As noted already, approaches to policy are many and varied. One method of organizing these differences is shown in Table 2.1, which illustrates the theoretical basis of approaches to policy, not the more obvious methods and prescriptions, and thus exposes more of the underlying differences and linkages across disciplines, political ideologies and policy preferences.

Table 2.1 *Approaches to policy and politics*

Unit of analysis	*Method of theory construction*	
	Deductive	**Inductive**
Individual	Rational choice theories (public choice)	Sociological individualism (welfare economics)
Collective or group	Class analysis (Marxism)	Group theories (pluralism/corporatism)
Structure (institutions)	Actor-centred institutionalism (transaction cost analysis)	Neo-institutionalism (statism)

Source: adapted from Howlett and Ramesh (2003, p22)

Deductive approaches apply general theories (and often generalized solutions) across specific cases. Inductive approaches distil insights from specific cases and are wary of generalizing these. For example, public choice is an approach utilized mostly by economists, a discipline that attaches great emphasis to the 'invisible hand' theory where individual expression of choices through markets is a fundamental social force and prime policy lever (e.g. Gillroy and Wade, 1992). This approach usually recommends markets or prices as mechanisms of influence. Approaches in the pluralism/corporatism category – often employed by political scientists – examine the interactions of groups in actual situations and tend not to offer recommendations for policy prescriptions. Here we can see that policy recommendations do not necessarily or even usually reflect an 'objective' stance, but rather are influenced by underlying assumptions and preferences.

Can policy be rational?

If the 'rational comprehensive' approach to policy is unrealistic and too demanding on time and information, how 'rational' can policy analysis and policy-making be, and what is the role of idealized 'models' of the policy process? To state that in politics and policy everything is contingent, contested and variable according to the context may be true, but is unhelpful in a practical sense to people who wish to understand or make better policy. Some reasonably well-structured description – that is, a model of some kind – of how policy can be understood is surely needed. Similarly, 'incrementalism' may be an accurate description of reality, but may not be helpful in thinking about how things could happen, and more structured models have valuable analytical uses (Dye, 1983). In the next chapter, we will present two such models – one developed in a public policy tradition, one developed from emergency

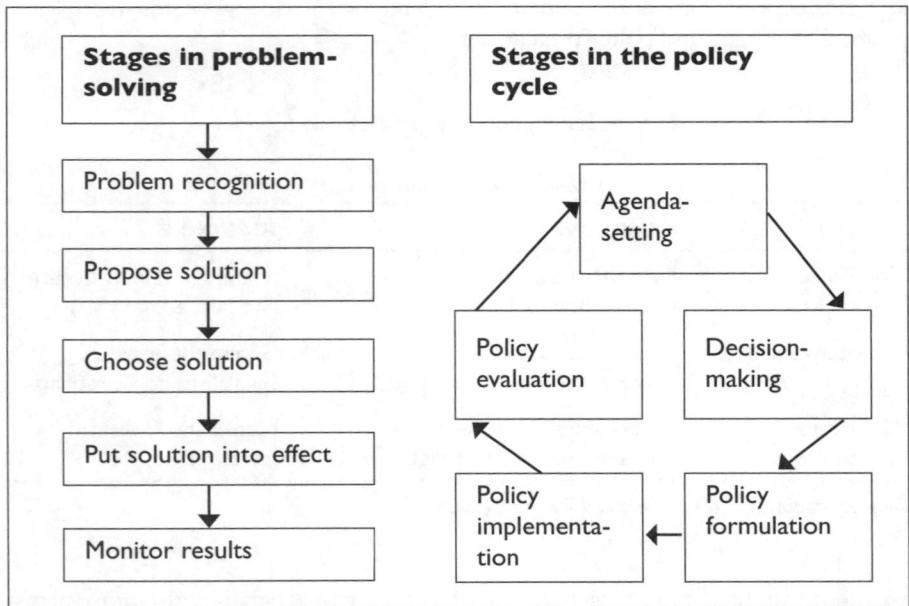

Figure 2.1 *Linear versus cyclic constructions of policy*

Source: adapted from Howlett and Ramesh (2003)

management – and use them to inform a consolidated framework and to structure later chapters. Here, we will simply mention some major kinds of models of the policy process, noting their strengths and dangers.

Before this, note that although strict sequential descriptions of how policy decisions should be made are somewhat unfashionable in recent writings on public policy, many policy officials and emergency (and other) managers are increasingly bound to follow tight standards and procedures, such as those developed for quality assurance, risk assessment or environmental management. Do the standards and procedures required of professional managers, imposed in an age of accountability and efficiency, signal a return to the rational comprehensive ideal?

Few texts in modern public policy follow a rational comprehensive approach, although many scientists, activists and members of the public appear to believe that a clear and linear process *should* exist. Most texts do, however, utilize some form of model of the policy process to illustrate the main aspects or stages, and then explain the complexity and variability of those elements. Figure 2.1 shows, side by side, the key elements of a linear problem-solving approach and a simplified policy cycle model. The main features are not dissimilar; but two key differences exist. One is the emphasis on the iterative and cyclical nature of policy, and the other is the explicit recognition that one might enter the cycle at any stage.

The examples in Figure 2.1 summarize many models of the policy process. Questions arise over how to choose and assess the usefulness of any given model. First, the choice of a model describing the policy process will, to a greater or lesser extent (depending on the model), determine the questions asked, methods used and information sought. Any model has a theoretical, conceptual or philosophical basis, so we need to be clear what that is. A focus on individual choice may ignore institutions and human behaviours not based on maximizing economic utility; an institutional focus may err in the reverse direction. It is dangerous to see a model of the policy process as a representation of either how the world works or how it should work. Similarly dangerous is to ignore the complexity of what lies beneath a simple description of a policy stage, such as 'problem recognition' or 'policy implementation'. The applicability of a general model to a specific domain may also be questionable – the problem context is important. This is especially the case with emergencies and disasters, for reasons given later in this chapter.

In response to these dangers, we propose four principles:

1 Be clear about the underlying assumptions of a policy model.
2 Make explicit the heuristic value of models and warn against assuming them to be definitive or prescriptive.
3 Recognize the detailed tasks and challenges lurking within summary stages.
4 Translate and adapt a model to the specific policy domain, where necessary (in the case of emergencies, this refers especially to the inherent unpredictability that will disturb any step-wise model).

This is done in Chapter 3, where we propose and explain two related frameworks/models for describing, analysing and, if not prescribing then at least suggesting, emergency and disaster policy.

Defining problems and solutions

If a problem is wrongly stated, then the solution to that problem (a policy intervention) will only be effective by sheer luck. Dery (1984) speaks of applying 'pseudo-solutions' to 'pseudo-problems'. Perhaps surprisingly, the policy literature lacks useful typologies of policy problems that extend beyond simple categories and classifications (Linder and Peters, 1989). A key to problem definition is to separate *substantive issues* (e.g. vulnerability to wildfire) from the *policy problems* that these present (e.g. land-use planning and encouraging changes in housing design). Later in this chapter, as a first step in a more careful definition of policy problems, we identify the *specific attributes* of policy problems in emergencies and disasters in order to clarify the features of these problems, rendering them different or difficult, and to consider what this means for policy responses (further explored in Chapters 5 and 6). Recognition of the preconditions for better problem definition is built into the frameworks presented in Chapter 3. Importantly, this will include recognition and discussion of the question of *who gets to define problems*, a necessarily value-laden and political topic, but one that cannot be ignored.

Choosing the 'solution' to the problem – *policy instrument choice* – is too often undertaken on the basis of convenience, expediency or disciplinary or ideological bias. Single instruments are often advocated in a general sense, when typically a mixture suited to specific contexts will be needed. Detailed menus of all possible instruments are often not considered or compared against rigorous criteria. Strangely, in the policy literature, there is no consensus on how to choose the best instrument or even agreement on what the options are (Linder and Peters, 1989; Howlett, 1991). This is, in part, due to the difficulty of being prescriptive across widely varying policy domains. In Chapter 6, the policy instruments will be addressed in greater detail in a manner specific to emergencies and disasters.

Information, learning and policy

One would expect it to be commonplace that we learn from policy experience and build lessons in a proactive way in order to get better at 'doing' policy. Yet, it appears that this is not often enough the case. On the basis of long experience, Lee (1993, p185) stated that 'deliberate learning is possible, though surely uncommon, in public policy'. This is an unacceptable situation, especially in an area such as emergencies and disasters, where the stakes are high and opportunities to learn limited and difficult. As many authors state, learning must entail improved understanding and capacities, not straight transfer or mimicry (May, 1992; Rose, 2005). May (1992) provides a typology: instrumental learning by officials and others regarding specific instruments or programme design; social learning about the construction of policy problems and goals, and the scope of policy; and political learning where actors gain knowledge about policy processes and how to advance their case. We will explore this issue in the emergencies context in Chapter 7.

The role of information in policy is an ongoing matter of debate (see Lindblom and Cohen, 1979). Contemporary understanding of policy processes recognizes multiple forms of information feeding into policy-making, from within government, the community, media and 'expert' sources, such as research organizations and individual scientists. Knowledge-based communities (known as 'epistemic communities') can play a crucial role in influencing policy; but those with formal expertise may not recognize the validity of 'non-expert' knowledge – such as the views of people potentially affected by a flood who disagree with the experts' probability estimate. The rational comprehensive or linear view of policy-making is unsettled by multiple inputs of information from multiple and very different knowledge systems. Information in policy processes is neither simple nor value free: different groups have divergent views of what is important, assumptions about how policy should function, and claims and rejections of the validity of knowledge. These may equal radically different rationalities gathered into a number of conflicting 'discourses' around the interaction between human and natural systems (Dryzek, 1997). With emergencies and disasters, there is a particularly wide catchment of relevant knowledge: various natural and social sciences, agencies and individuals directly involved, the private sector, non-government players such as charities and professional groups, and local communities. Across and even within each, knowledge will be diverse and contested, and pity the policy-makers who must reconcile expectations and produce a fair and effective outcome. The role of information, and how we learn from it, will be revisited in this book.

The role of government

Government is the central actor in public policy, even when non-government players and communities play strong roles also. Yet, 'government' is a vague term, shorthand for the state sector and public bodies. Accurately, government is the administration in power in a jurisdiction, representative of one or more political parties in a legislature. Systems of public administration vary across jurisdictions. Table 2.2 identifies the key components of government systems that play a role in policy processes.

In any specific situation, making sense of policy is not possible without accuracy regarding the relevant landscape of government and public administration at a finer resolution than depicted in Table 2.2 in terms of structure and function – that is, what the parts are called, but also what activities they undertake and in what fashion. In a cross-sectoral policy domain, such as emergencies and disasters, at any given time, more than one of these components will be actively involved in various aspects of the policy process. Increasingly recognized as being of particular importance are the roles of informal and institutional arrangements at local scales, generally and especially in policy domains such as disasters where achievement of stated goals will depend on collaboration with affected communities. Chapter 8 explores in more detail the actual and potential roles of different components in framing institutional responses to emergencies and disasters.

Thus far, we have noted that ideologies, disciplinary assumptions and so on are important in policy-making, as much as objective and rational methods or processes. That is neither bad nor avoidable, as Davis et al (1993, p257) remind us:

> Politics is *the* essential ingredient for producing workable policies, which are more publicly accountable and politically justifiable... While some are uncomfortable with the notion that politics can enhance rational decision-making, preferring to see politics as expediency, it is integral to the process of securing defensible outcomes. We are unable to combine values, interests and resources in ways which are not political.

Table 2.2 Key components of the governing state

Head of state	Head of government (e.g. president) or separate (e.g. monarch or president, with government led by prime minister)
Legislature (national or state/provincial)	The parliament, parliamentary committees, etc.
Executive	Leader of government (president, prime minister, premier), cabinet, ministers/secretaries, government and ministerial staff
Public service departments	Line departments and central agencies (e.g. treasury, health, transport, defence, etc).
Statutory authorities	More independent than departments, such as national parks services, emergency services authorities, research and statistical bureaus, intelligence agencies, etc.
Judicial and regulatory bodies	High or supreme courts, lesser courts, specific bodies (e.g. consumer or monopolies commissions, etc.)
Enforcement agencies	Police customs services
Local government	Variable in size, independence, roles and powers across jurisdictions
Intergovernmental bodies	National-state/provincial joint bodies (e.g. ministerial councils, inter-jurisdictional river basin organizations, standard-setting boards, national advisory councils, etc.)
Public trading corporations	Government-controlled bodies (e.g. broadcasting corporations, power and water utilities, etc.)
'Semi-state institutions', private bodies and NGOs	Unions, churches, universities, charities, political parties, etc. who play an organized role in policy debates or implementation
Informal and community institutions	Volunteer groups, communal associations, kin and other networks, etc.

Source: adapted from Davis et al (1993)

Politics is about reconciling or arguing over different values in society, and about the distribution of costs and benefits, whether these are economic or otherwise. Policy is how politics does things, so policy is political. This is rarely more the case than with emergencies and disasters, where the costs and benefits may be literally, life and death, or at least livelihood or no livelihood, a comfortable existence or constant dislocation. Politics and values cannot be avoided in policy, and certainly should never be ignored. This makes understanding and (even more) influencing policy much more complex; but we can at least identify some of the big political ideas and trends within which a policy domain such as emergencies and disasters exists.

Policy styles and the political environment

Emergency management approaches are influenced – whether enabled or constrained – by surrounding policy processes and institutional systems. These, in turn, reflect the broad policy styles adopted by government and society, and also by interaction with other big political trends and ideas. Human safety and protection of livelihoods from disasters is but one political and social goal: there are others, often more powerful, or at least vying for discussion space, resources and priority.

Different political and social goals and trends may interact in a synergistic fashion or in opposition, or in ways that are more complex and difficult to discern. Here, we will briefly consider three political trends and ideas (globalization, neo-liberalism and participatory democracy) and two other major issues (sustainability and security), and the ways in which they interact with emergencies and disasters.

Globalization is an oft-used term with multiple meanings (Stiglitz, 2002). It captures a suite of related phenomenon, involving global financial and commercial interdependency, the internationalization of political discussion, laws and policies, media, images and ideas, and the movement of goods, services and people. National state boundaries and the natural isolation of communities no longer insulate people, communities or economies as they once did from events and changes elsewhere. As we state in Chapter 1, the impacts of disasters are now better known and felt across borders than once they were. Responses to disasters may be swifter and more effective with information and transport flow in a global world, and via international agreements and obligations. Preparation and warning may be similarly enhanced, enabled by flows of information, technology and expertise. Conversely, local communities may be made more rather than less vulnerable to disasters by diminished economic and social resilience arising from increased dependence on single commodity production in a competitive global economic system, or by capital flight in responsive global financial markets.

Related to economic globalization is the powerful impact of neo-liberal political thought, neoclassical economic theory and the practical manifestations of these (see Gilroy and Wade, 1992; Stiglitz, 2002). At root, this favours private-sector and market-based policy styles and instruments rather than traditional government-led approaches. This is argued on the basis of efficiency, and emphasis is placed on the power and validity of individual choice in competitive markets as a basis for social choice. Such political thinking has led to the promotion of market-based policy instruments, privatization and the corporatization of public services (e.g. water and energy supply, welfare and health services), outsourcing of functions, and a diminishing of the capacities and size of the state. Related is the trend known as new public management (NPM), where client focus, efficiency in delivery, leanness in organizations and devolution of functions are emphasized (see McLaughlin et al, 2002). Generic management principles gain ascendancy over sector-specific traditions. Due to its history (see Chapter 1) and the public good nature of the enterprise in the emergency and disaster area, this has had less impact than in some other policy sectors. Nonetheless, NPM has affected many individual agencies; privatization and corporation of functions (e.g. in the health system and in remote sensing) are relevant to emergencies and disasters; and there is increased interest in market instruments in disaster prevention (e.g. insurance, financial incentives and disincentives for building practices, etc.).

Running somewhat counter to the neo-liberal trend is increasing interest in, and demands for, more participatory democracy and policy-making, often discussed under the titles of deliberative or discursive democracy (Dryzek, 2000; Dobson, 2003; Fisher, 2003; Fung and Wright, 2003). Critics see this move as largely rhetorical and point to a lack of change in actual political structures; others see a rise of civil society movements and the use of more inclusive processes in some jurisdictions. The shift in emergency management towards more community-based approaches is consistent in tone (and sometimes in style) with the arguments for participatory approaches. This is explored further in Chapter 4.

Sustainability is a major political and social agenda, emphasizing the long-run viability of human societies in the face of declining natural resources and increasingly stressed environments, and links this environmental agenda to human development in both social and economic terms (see Lafferty and Meadowcroft, 2000; Berkhout et al, 2002; Connor and Dovers, 2004; Elliott, 2005). The emphasis is on the integration of environmental, social and economic concerns in policy; precaution in the face of uncertainty; the long-term, inclusive and innovative approaches to policy-making and implementation; and the protection of ecological functions that underpin human societies. Sustainability thus has many shared concerns with emergencies and disasters (and might even be construed as subsuming disasters as a policy agenda), and many international agreements and processes, and much literature, link the two closely. The two policy areas do interact, both synergistically and with tension (Dovers, 2004). In management terms, some emergency management practices may conflict with environmental conservation, such as modification of riparian areas for floodwater egress. Yet, in other ways, sustainability and disasters have similar aims and, thus, potentially similar policy strategies, such as increasing resilience and diversity in local communities and their links with their environment.

In recent years, especially since the terrorist attacks of 11 September 2001, issues of 'national security' and the 'war on terror' have risen to dominate political and policy agendas. This has impacted profoundly on political styles, global alliances of nations, the availability of information, and on the public and political space available for other issues. Regardless of the validity of the national security agenda, we simply note that the direct human and economic costs of terrorism are insignificant compared to more familiar natural and technological disasters. Yet, security absorbs more financial, legal and human resources, shifts public and political attention away from other issues, and appears to have diverted some emergency management capacity.

As an aside, the rise of information and communication technology (ICT) could be categorized as another major trend or issue, and has transformed, or is transforming, the potential and practice of many sectors, including emergencies and disasters. Here, though, we will treat ICT as an enabling and interacting factor relating to trends such as globalization and participation.

Considering these three trends and two issues, two critical considerations emerge. The first is to recognize the important and often complex interaction between these trends and issues, and their effect on emergency and disaster policy and management. The second is to be sensitive to the way in which these interactions, and the priority given to particular ideas, manifest in different cultures, countries and political and legal settings. Different countries evidence quite different 'policy styles' – general attitudes towards the who, how and why of policy-making – related to ideas such as individual rights, democracy, the role of the state versus the market, and so on. Some countries tend towards government provision of services and regulation, others towards a more market-based system. Some countries formulate policy and construct and run institutions in an inclusive manner; some include only major interest groups ('corporatism'); whereas in other agencies of the state, the executive itself is the key player.

Yet, it is very rare that any country or jurisdiction relies only on one policy style; rather, different styles are used in various mixtures, and these change over time (as circumstances or governments change) and, importantly, across issues. This point is especially relevant to emergencies and disasters where, given the potentially extreme costs of getting it wrong, the choice of policy style should relate closely to the precise nature of the policy problem. This is pursued further in Chapters 6 and 8.

A further point is the ability to learn across jurisdictions, cultures and policy styles and instruments. In a policy area where the costs of failure may be catastrophic, and where the ability to 'experiment' is limited, there is a strong imperative to gain lessons and insights from other places, and thus to engage in comparative policy analysis, an issue discussed above. The intent of analysis is not to copy across contexts, but to learn (Rose, 2005). This is discussed in Chapter 7.

This section makes it clear that the problems faced in emergencies and disasters are multiple, complex and vary greatly in magnitude. We now turn to ways that attempt to render this confusing suite of problems more comprehensible.

Emergencies and disasters as policy and institutional problems

The various ways in which emergencies and disasters are defined were canvassed in Chapter 1. Clearly, by definition, emergencies and disasters challenge policy processes and the actors, organizations and institutions that shape policy. Boin et al (2005, pix) state this sharply:

> Crises make and break political careers, shake bureaucratic pecking orders and shape organizational destinies. Crises fix the spotlight on those who govern. Heroes and villains emerge with a speed and intensity quite unknown to 'politics as usual'.

It only takes a brief reflection on tsunamis, floods or earthquakes to define disasters as very difficult policy problems. Yet, it helps to delve deeper into this, and to isolate the main attributes of emergencies and disasters that serve to make them different and difficult as problems for policy and institutional systems.[2] The following attributes characterize emergencies and disasters, and can assist in framing policy responses:

- *Spatial and temporal scales*, respectively, are broader and lengthier than those characterizing most policy challenges. The spatial extent of emergencies generally fits poorly with the political and administrative boundaries within which much information and policy is organized. Likewise, the occurrence (and non-occurrence) of disasters in time, and their long-lived legacies, do not match electoral or budget cycles and, hence, the time scales of normal political, administrative and economic decision-making. The temporal scale of disasters has two contrasting characteristics: long periods demanding preparedness that may be difficult to justify, and rapid onset events that entail sudden impacts and enormous political urgency.
- *Magnitude and stakes*: here the prospect – and sometimes reality – of disasters is that they may literally destroy communities. This poses the prospect of irreversible impacts and irreversible implications of policy decisions, and, thus, a much lower opportunity at times to learn from experience.
- *Multiple and interactive causes* involve two dimensions. The first is multiple causes that do not operate in isolation, such as natural phenomena and human actions causing vulnerability at their intersection. Second, while the *direct* causes of emergencies and disasters (e.g. a wildfire or a chemical spill) are important, in a policy sense the *indirect* causes may be better targets for proactive policy response (e.g. dysfunctional land-use planning or poor compliance with technical standards).
- There is a strong need for the *participation* of a wide range of actors in both policy and management, including governments, research bodies, local communities and NGOs. Traditional reliance on government action has been replaced with a reliance on multiple partnerships and cooperation.
- *Pervasive risk and uncertainty* exists, including uncertainty as to the timing, location and magnitude of events, but equally about the efficacy of human comprehension, vulnerability and coping capacity.
- *Moral dimensions* are significant due to the frequent need for assistance from other communities or nations in times of crisis, including decisions as to the contribution of negligence by affected communities and their governments. *Multiple values* exist where values are perceived differently by varying groups in society (e.g. human lives and livelihoods, emotional trauma, economic sectors, cultural integrity and environmental values).
- *Non-marketed assets* are difficult to value economically and thus enter into dominant ideas of cost-benefit in protection or recovery. Similarly, in emergency and disasters, there is typically a challenging mixture of public and private costs and benefits, raising issues of responsibility.
- *Poorly defined policy rights and responsibilities*: while understandable given the uncertainty and complexity of emergencies and disasters, it is apparent that the assignment of roles and responsibilities for understanding, preparing for and

responding to events is often unclear. This is particularly the case when it comes to addressing the underlying causes of disasters.

Taken in combination, these attributes confirm that emergencies and disasters are big, complex and, indeed, both difficult and different. While other policy domains and problems are not 'easy', they rarely have multiple combinations of these attributes. The critically important point that emerges is that given the nature of emergencies and disasters, it is likely that existing policy and institutional capacities, which have co-evolved with such other policy domains, creating the traditions and trends summarized above, can reasonably be expected to struggle with emergencies and disasters. So, while standard policy thinking has much to offer this domain (and, we argue, has not sufficiently in the past), caution must be exercised in drawing lessons from it. If emergencies and disasters are significantly different in kind, then it follows that the necessary policy and institutional responses will also be different. Given that disasters are abnormal by definition, this is an obvious point, perhaps; but it has not often enough been used in a structured way to explore policy and institutional responses, as is the aim of this book.

Chapter 5 delves deeper into the issue of problem framing and, drawing on these attributes, sets out a three-category classification of emergencies and disasters.

Reconciling policy with emergencies and disasters

This chapter has identified some central concepts and realities that have captured the attention and effort of the discipline and profession of public policy for many years. The terms 'policy' and 'institutions' are complex and contested, and the issue of policy and institutional settings to handle emergencies and disasters has been presented as doubly so.

The focus of this book is on the broader issue of policy processes operating within institutional systems, more than on organizational details or particular policy instruments and the outcomes of applying them. The next chapter will present two models. It will explain the detailed challenges, seeking to do justice to, first, what we know (and do not know) about policy, and, second, what we know (and do not know) about the nature of emergencies and disasters. From these two models, a new framework is presented to inform description, analysis and prescription of policy and institutional responses to emergencies and disasters. Later chapters will go into particular elements of that framework in more detail, not seeking to prescribe precise choices, but to identify the range of options, how they can be compared and their relative merits under different circumstances.

Notes

1   This set of definitions is consistent with those in Dovers (2005). They vary from, but are not inconsistent with, terminology used in other literature; for discussions, see, for example, North (1990), Goodin (1996), Howlett and Ramesh (2003) and Connor and Dovers (2004).

2   This set of attributes follows one developed for sustainability problems, a problem domain closely related to emergencies and disasters (see Dovers, 1997, 2005).

Part II

Constructing the Response

3

A Policy and Institutional Framework for Emergencies and Disasters

This chapter draws on Chapter 1, which explored the nature of emergencies and disasters, and on Chapter 2, which examined the nature of policy and institutions. It combines these insights to create a framework for describing, analysing and prescribing broad approaches to policy and institutional settings for emergencies and disasters. It considers the suitability of the standard policy cycle model approach and an emergency risk management framework; assesses their strengths and gaps; and develops a new framework specifically designed to address emergencies and disasters, and to better address the strategic policy and institutional perspective that is the focus of this book. Key elements of the framework are explored in more detail in later chapters.

Policy cycles meet emergency risk management

As we saw in Chapter 2, models and characterizations of policy processes are to be treated with care; however, they are very useful tools to structure and make more comprehensive the description, analysis and (with even greater care) prescription of policy. They are also often generic and simple – applying the same thinking and concepts to any policy sector and categorizing a small number of 'stages' in the policy process. A little later we will present a *framework* (rather than a model) that is considerably more detailed, and which is better suited to a policy sector characterized by complexity and uncertainty, such as emergencies and disasters. It also pays more attention to what happens before and after the 'policy', and to general principles that should inform policy-making and the institutional settings within which policy is made. It was developed specifically for the not dissimilar domain of environment and sustainability, drawing on traditional public policy literature and practice (see Figure 3.1(a)). The choice of environment and sustainability as a domain for lesson drawing is based on shared problem attributes with emergencies and disasters: policy challenges arising at the intersection of natural and human systems; extended spatial and temporal scales; complexity and connectivity; pervasive uncertainty; demands and justification for community participation; ill-defined policy and property rights; and so on.

In Chapter 1, we observed that the bulk of thinking to do with disasters has – often with very positive impact – largely concerned emergency *management*, focusing on the operational challenges of preparedness, response and recovery. While vitally necessary, here we wish to extend thinking more towards the policy processes and institutional settings within which emergency and disaster management operates, and to expand and detail the array of actors involved. As a starting point, we consider an expanded version of the Emergency Risk Management (ERM) framework developed in Australia from the internationally regarded Australian–New Zealand Risk Management Standard (EMA, 2000; Standards Australia, 2004) (see Figure 3.1(b)). As explained below, the extended framework expands the scope of traditional emergency management thinking to incorporate considerations essential to the intent and scope of this book.

The two frameworks in Figure 3.1 provide a detailed basis for considering the key issues for policy and institutional development in emergencies and disasters. They allow us not to simply contain the drawing of insights and lessons from one field or perspective, but from multiple sources that are relevant. The basis of each – traditional public policy and traditional emergency management – however, is not fully sufficient, as the frameworks still do not cover some aspects that Chapters 1 and 2 identified as critically important. The following are not so much criticisms of public policy and emergency management as statements of understandable limitation, recognizing that, when combined, these two frameworks may offer more:

- Traditional policy cycles are focused on *public* policy – that is, on the actions and imperatives of government. They tend to compress the problem-framing dimension of policy to the appearance of issues on the government agenda, downplay the complexity and dynamics of non-government interests, fail to consider institutional aspects in sufficient detail, and ignore uncertainty. They are also generic, and inevitably require adjustment to the specific character of policy sectors and substantive issues where they might be applied. The framework summarized in Figure 3.1(a) addresses such shortcomings in the context of interactions between human and natural systems (where both disasters and issues of sustainability arise), and extending more into the complex realm of problem framing.
- Traditional emergency management focuses on precisely that: operational issues and procedures of *management*. The Emergency Risk Management (ERM) process is, in many people's view, an improvement on the preparedness–response–recovery conceptualization, but nonetheless similarly downplays matters such as residual uncertainty, problem framing, strategic policy choice and coordination, and organizational and institutional settings. The extended ERM process summarized in Figure 3.1(b) explicitly incorporates these considerations.

Even so, neither framework in Figure 3.1 is by itself sufficient, not surprisingly as both have been developed for purposes different than that here. For example, the policy framework has less attention placed on the crucial issue of risk and uncertainty, whereas the extended ERM process overlooks policy framing and implementation. However, in combination, they cover a wide range of elements of a potential guiding framework for considering policies and institutions for emergencies and disasters.

In policy processes: general elements – coordination/integration, communication, participation, transparency and accountability

In institutional settings: general elements – persistence, purposefulness, information richness, inclusiveness and flexibility

Problem framing and agenda-setting:
* negotiation of social goals;
* monitoring of linked natural–human systems;
* identification of problematic change;
* identification of direct and underlying causes;
* assessment of uncertainty;
* assessment of other policy settings;
* definition of policy problems.

Policy framing and strategic choice:
* identification of policy principles;
* strategic policy choices (policy style);
* definition of policy goals.

Policy design and implementation:
* selection of policy instruments;
* planning implementation, information and communication;
* resource provision (statutory, information, institutional, financial);
* enforcement/compliance mechanisms;
* establishment of policy monitoring and review processes.

Policy monitoring and evaluation:
* ongoing policy monitoring and routine data capture;
* mandated evaluation process;
* extension, adaptation or cessation of policy and/or goals.

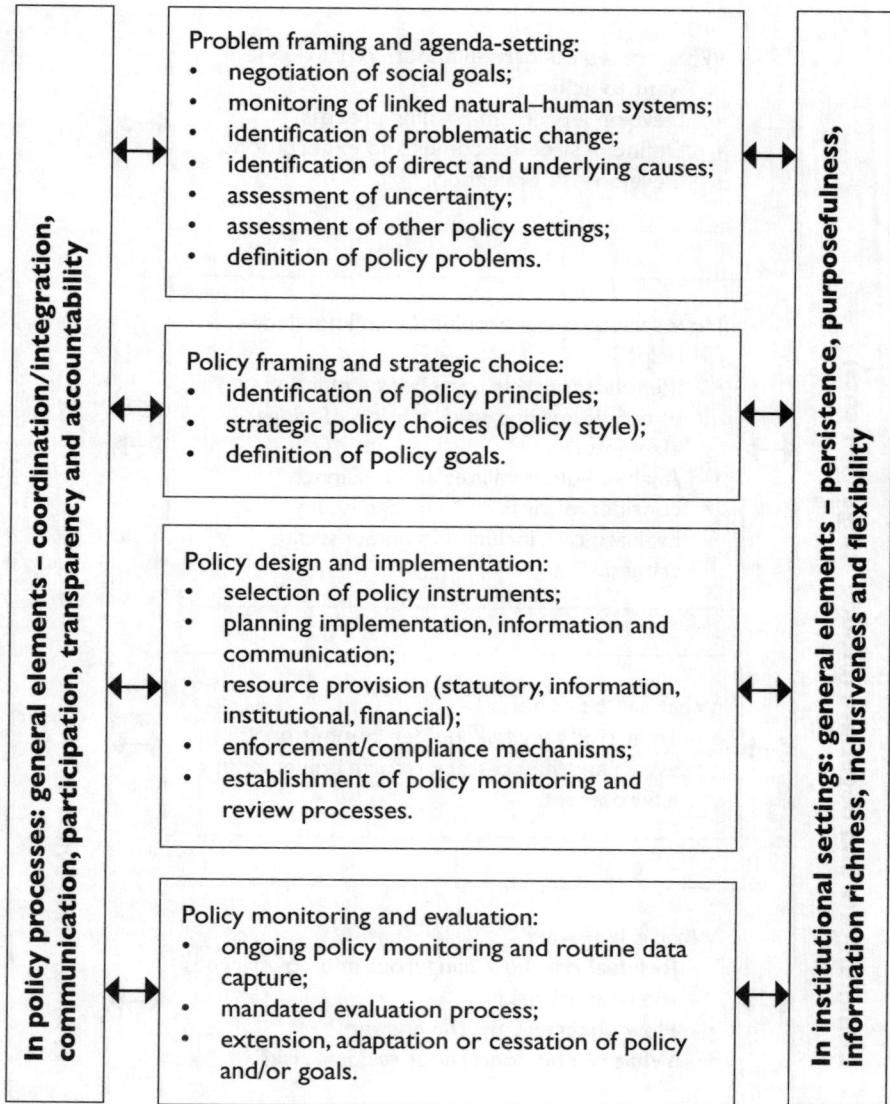

Figure 3.1 *(a) Framework for environment and sustainability policy*

Source: (a) Dovers (2005), drawing on Howlett and Ramesh (2003), Bridgman and Davis (2004) and other sources

What are we concerned about? What do we
    want to achieve?
- Develop a problem-framing process.
- Define desired outcomes and expectations.
- Develop risk evaluation.

How serious is the problem? Can knowledge
    help?
- Identification: this comprises a plurality
    of definitions and the inclusion of fringe
    elements.
- Analyse vulnerabilities and resilience;
    consider fairness and outrage issues.
- Evaluate risk: include incommensurate
    criteria.

What can be done?
- Treat risk: gain stakeholder commitment;
    assess and, if necessary, reform implementing
    environment.

What is left over?
- Residual risk: how dangerous and how large is
    the residual risk?
- How uncertain are the answers?
- What can be done about residual risk?

Communicate and negotiate (include fringe elements)

Monitor and review

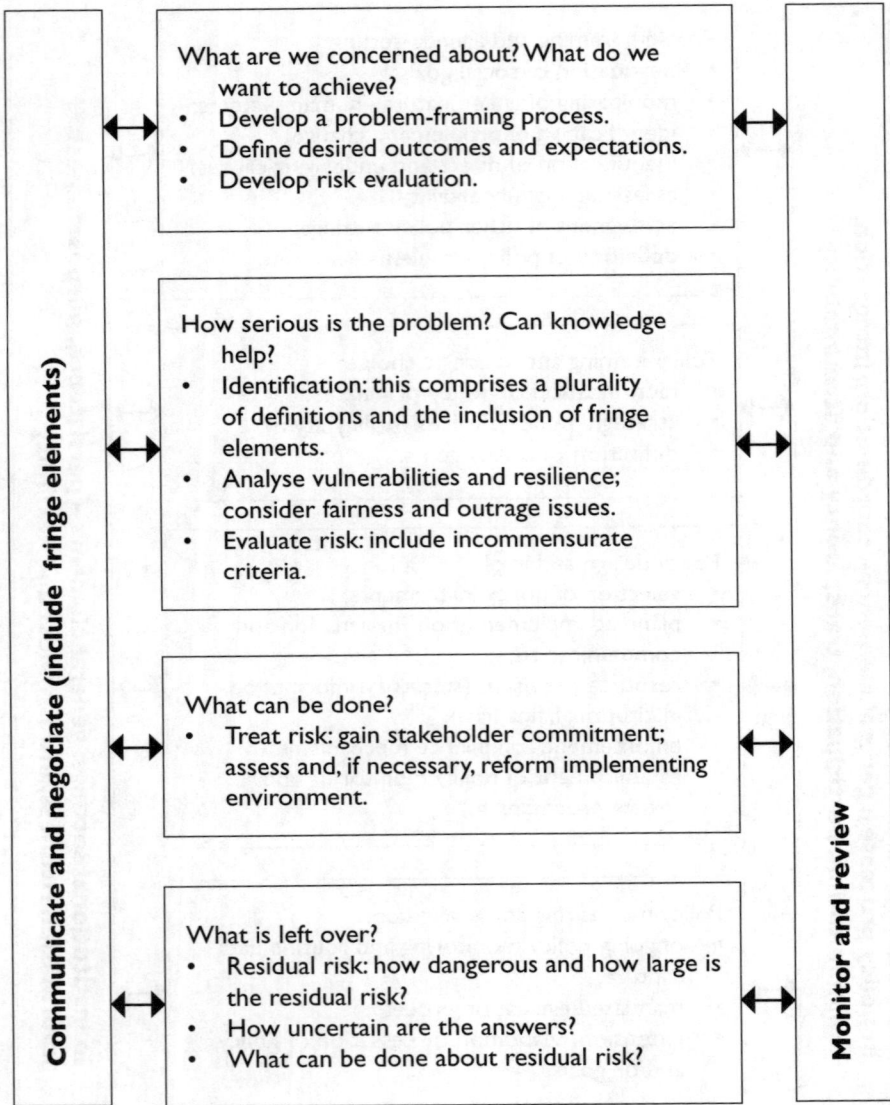

Figure 3.1 *(b) The extended emergency risk management process*

Source: (b) adapted from the Australian Emergency Risk Management Standard (EMA, 2000) and an extended Post-Normal Science version (Funtowicz and Ravetz, 1993;[1] Handmer and Proudley, 2005)

We also need to be cognizant of the key themes that were identified in Chapter 1, such as the:

- whole-of-society and whole-of-government nature of emergencies and disasters, when considering causes, impacts and responsibilities;
- critical role that community vulnerability and, conversely, resilience play in defining the possibility and impacts of emergencies and disasters;
- importance of how emergencies and disasters are framed as policy and institutional problems, not only as 'events';
- necessity of incorporating explicit consideration of residual risk and uncertainty in framing policy and designing institutions;
- need for long-term (strategic) policy development, as well as event- and response-focused policy settings;
- need for more structured and detailed processes for policy instrument choice and policy implementation;
- importance of learning across time and place, and the connection of this to adaptive processes;
- necessity of considering redundancy and non-optimized capacities in the face of large-scale potential impacts;
- crucial role that broader institutional factors play in all of the above.

These key challenges, which represent more cross-cutting issues, together with the frameworks depicted in Figure 3.1, provide the basis for the integrated framework presented in the next section.

A framework for policy and institutional analysis

The framework set out in this section combines an understanding of both policy and disasters. Figure 3.2 presents a framework for emergencies and disasters policy and institutional analysis that incorporates key elements of the two perspectives summarized in Figure 3.1. It does not say 'how' to design policies and institutions, but rather gathers together critical elements and considerations that, if carefully considered and acted on as appropriate in a given situation, will significantly increase the likelihood of designing effective and comprehensive policy and institutional responses. In other words, Figure 3.2 represents a comprehensive and integrated *framework and checklist*, not a prescriptive model or sequence. The lines between the elements of the framework recognize that, while neither in theory nor in practice strictly a cycle, the elements are nonetheless tightly interdependent. It may be utilized in whole or in part, and at any given time and place an individual or organization may be situated or interested in different stages. However, it is in its entirety that the framework is most powerful as a prompt to understanding and considering the interrelated nature of policy and institutional responses to emergencies and disasters.

The following describes in summary form the main stages and subsidiary elements of the framework, all of which are expanded on in later chapters:

- *Problem framing (stage 1).* This stage emphasizes the importance of how we arrive at an understanding of policy and institutional problems in emergencies and disasters. Damaging events or natural phenomena such as floods are not policy or institutional problems, but they serve to define such problems, along with the characteristics of human systems. Problem framing can simply involve the decisions of elites and experts, or other subsets of the community. But we argue that it is better to construe problem framing as including episodes of social debate and ongoing discourse between parts of the community; ongoing monitoring and knowledge generation; the identification of direct and indirect causes of vulnerability and resilience; assessment of other supportive or constraining policy and institutional settings; and the open assessment of risk and uncertainty. A more realistic, tractable and widely understood definition of the policy problem emerges from the combination of those elements.
- *Policy framing and strategic policy choice (stage 2).* The policy response of a society or a government can be reactive and not openly informed by multiple perspectives. Or it can be more proactive, involving the clear choice of general policy styles (coercive, community oriented, market based, etc.), based on clearly understood principles and aimed at achieving agreed and clear objectives. Policy styles and goals in the disasters field should explicitly address conflicting or minority concerns and the situations of marginalized groups. Strategic policy choice defines the parameters and directions within which later policy design and implementation occur – that is, what and who is included and excluded – and thus is a crucial point in the policy process.
- *Policy design and implementation (stage 3).* Ideally, achieving policy objectives involves the choice of specific policy instruments chosen transparently from a wide menu of options. To implement these instruments, resources are required (financial, informational, human, administrative, statutory, etc.). Some degree of enforcement or compliance will often be necessary, and mechanisms for ongoing monitoring should be put in place to allow later evaluation, learning and adaptation.
- *Policy monitoring and learning (stage 4).* In an uncertain and changing world, learning from experience and ongoing adaptation and improvement are demanded, and this stage requires attention to policy monitoring well after initial policy design and implementation. This stage, which may last for many years, involves continuing observation and routine collection of requisite data. The link between this and stage 1 (monitoring of human and natural systems) begs the integration of policy and basic monitoring to enable separation of the impact of policy interventions and other variables. It involves a mandated ability to react to and learn from unexpected events, as well as to mount formal evaluation exercises and act upon the findings.

Above and beyond the four stages above, and the subsidiary elements within them, there are principles and imperatives, identified in Figure 3.2, that need to be constantly accounted for throughout any exercise of policy or institutional analysis or design:

1 Problem framing discourse	Social debate and wide ownership of problems Ongoing monitoring, research and development, and inclusive discourse Identification of direct and underlying causes Identification of vulnerability/resilience, allowing multiple definitions and perceptions Assessment of uncertainty, including residual uncertainty And risk assessment procedures Definition of policy and institutional problems, including multiple interpretations
2 Policy framing and strategic policy choice	Choice of broad policy style/s Identification of relevant policy principles Definition of desired outcomes/policy goals Communication of policy statement/direction Assess other policies and institutional environment
3 Policy design and implementation	Policy instrument choice Implementation planning Provision of resources (multiple forms) Communication and information strategies Enforcement and compliance provisions Establishment of monitoring and adaptive learning mechanisms
4 Policy monitoring and learning	Ongoing monitoring and routine data capture Structured and adaptive learning from events Rigorous and mandated evaluation Adaptation, cessation, problem redefinition, etc.
Cross-cutting policy principles	Whole-of-government coordination Transparency and accountability Appropriate public participation
Institutional design imperatives	Coordination of actors and organizations Use of legal systems and instruments Clarity of roles and responsibilities Purposefulness and persistence over time Inclusion, especially of the less powerful Information richness and sensitivity Flexibility and adaptability

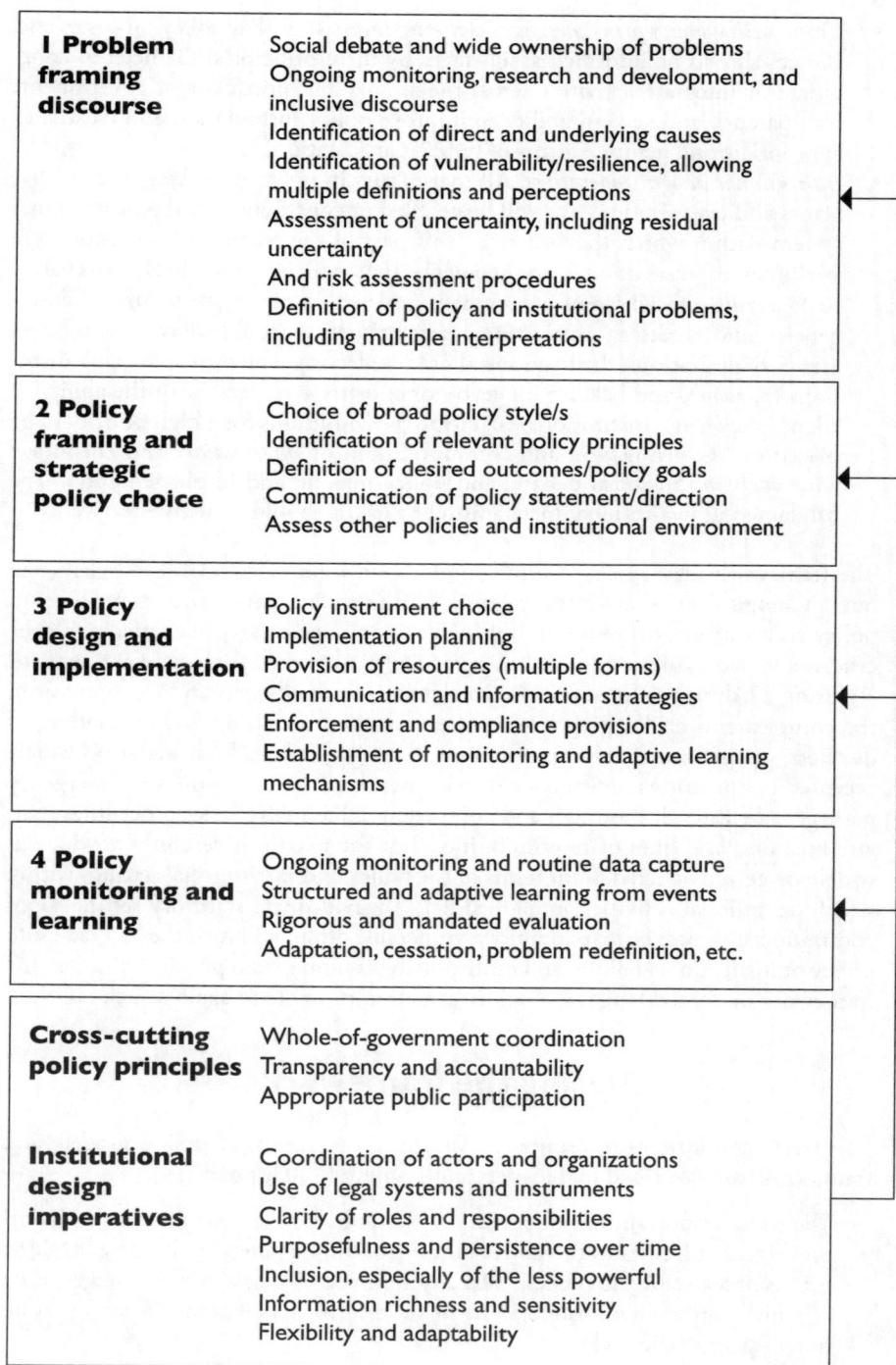

Figure 3.2 *Framework for policy and institutional analysis for emergencies and disasters*

- *Cross-cutting policy principles*. This element emphasizes that policy processes and choices should be informed at all stages by three principles: the need to coordinate or integrate activities across the sectors and portfolios of government; transparency and accountability to improve policy formulation and trust; and appropriate and genuine forms of public participation.
- *Institutional design imperatives*. All that occurs in policy processes, and all that actors and organizations do, will be enabled or constrained by the institutional system within which they operate. This part of the framework proposes core attributes of institutional arrangements that will be more likely to enable. Recognizing the whole-of-government and whole-of-society nature of emergencies and disasters, institutional arrangements should allow *coordination* across organizations. Institutions should reflect agreed principles and directions (*purpose*), and balance longevity of efforts (*persistence*) with the ability to adapt (*flexibility*). Institutions will create the conditions for a high priority to be placed on the acquisition and communication of *information*, and encourage wide *inclusion* in social debate, and policy-making and implementation. The fundamental institutional mechanism of the *law* should be used effectively.

The framework may appear overly complex – in total, it comprises 30 elements; but an honest and shared appreciation of the many things that contribute to policy and institutional response is valuable as any one or several elements may be crucial and too easily overlooked in a particular situation. A score of 90 per cent – getting 27 things right out of the 30 elements – usually gets an 'A' grade; but in the complex and challenging world of anticipating, preparing and responding to disasters, getting one thing wrong can cause terrible failure. That maxim is widely accepted in operational emergency management and is one reason why emergency managers are careful, thorough and competent, adhering to strict procedures, fail-safe measures and lines of responsibilities. But the maxim is certainly nowhere as widely perceived or acted on in terms of the policy and institutional settings within which operational activities are embedded. An inadequate statutory setting, poor communication or failure to identify a vulnerable group will turn the 'A' grade into policy or institutional failure, and quite possibly a human and political disaster. The framework presented here is a checklist, an attempt to guard against such failure.

Using the framework

The term 'checklist' is appropriate. The uses and limits of policy models and frameworks are described by Howlett and Ramesh (2003, pp13–14):

> The most important advantage of ... the policy cycle model as an analytical tool is that it facilitates the understanding of public policy-making by breaking the complexity of the process into any number of stages and sub-stages, each of which can be investigated alone or in terms of its relationship to any or all other stages of the cycle.

As noted in the previous chapter, there are those who are doubtful of the use of any form of model, believing the dangers of simplification and unthinking generic application outweigh the benefits. We would disagree; as long as strong qualifications are understood and maintained, a structured framework (especially a more comprehensive and context-sensitive one) is far better than none at all. The flexibility of having no model may make observation and *post-hoc* explanation possible; but for anyone interested in making the world less vulnerable to disasters, the absence of a model does not help much other than to produce a series of unconnected 'just-so stories'. A detailed framework suits the intent of this book and is also a structuring device: it helps to identify the many variables shaping policy and institutions, and to show why simplistic or partial interpretations and prescriptions are, by and large, not to be trusted in a complex world.

The following chapters explore in more detail the major elements of the framework:

- Chapter 4, 'Owning the problem', places the questions of community inclusion and public participation first and foremost, discussing the meaning of community, the purposes of participation, the role of communication in participation, and a variety of participatory strategies and techniques used or potentially valuable in emergency and disasters policy.
- Chapter 5, 'Framing the problem', deals with stage 1 of the framework, ranging across social and political debate, knowledge requirements, assessment of risk and uncertainty, and problem definition.
- Chapter 6, 'Responding to the problem', deals with stages 2 and 3 of the framework: the formulation and implementation of policy.
- Chapter 7, 'Not forgetting', deals with stage 4, covering the core considerations in policy monitoring and evaluation, and especially the higher-level issue of policy learning and change.
- Chapter 8, 'Institutional settings for emergencies and disasters', attends to what is perhaps the most often overlooked aspect of all – the institutional settings within which emergency policy and management happens, ranging from matters of organizational design to generic political and institutional challenges.
- In Chapter 9, 'Future prospects', we consider the prospects for improving societies' capacity to comprehend and cope with emergencies and disasters in the future, recognizing that while external variables play a role in creating vulnerability, the larger role – and one more in our realm of influence – will be played by our policies and institutions. The future should not be allowed to be only an accident.

Throughout the chapters, the general elements in the framework are incorporated and considered in terms of implementing these broad concerns within policy and institutional systems. In each chapter, the aim is to define the nature of each stage and element, and to identify key considerations and indicate options and approaches that may be put in place.

Given the enormous range of contexts in which these elements will have to be considered, the focus is on the interconnection of broader considerations and factors, not on recommending or designing specific policy and institutional strategies. The discussion avoids detailed, explanatory case studies. Such case studies would lengthen what is designed to be a reasonably short book, would inevitably only be relevant to a relatively few situations and would quickly date. Rather, we employ illustrative examples, including reference to the vignettes in Chapter 1, to ground the discussion and to demonstrate the relevance of the issues under discussion.

Note

1   Our thinking benefited from discussions with Bruna DeMarchi, Silvio Funtowicz, Jerry Ravetz, James Risbey and Jeroen van der Sluijs.

4

Owning the Problem: Politics, Participation and Communication

Chapters 1 and 3 emphasized the trend in policy, generally, and emergencies and disasters, in particular, to greater engagement with the 'community'. At a broader level, this shift (or proposed shift) is from government to governance; in more operational terms it is from top-down to community-oriented emergency management. Consistent with the argument that such engagement is crucial, we begin this part of the book with an examination of what this trend entails, to provide a clearer basis for considering options for more inclusive policy and institutional arrangements. As in the book as a whole, the focus is more on the policy and institutional level than on operational management. The chapter recalls and extends the discussion from Chapter 2 regarding the respective and varying roles of government, community and other players. It then goes beneath the general notion of 'community participation' to explore *the who, why and how of public participation*: defining community, the purposes of participation and forms of participation. Finally, the chapter discusses information and communication as central to participation.

Policy and politics

The engagement of citizens in the governance and policy-making of their society is an age-old and continuing question – why they should be engaged, concerning what issues and through what processes? Especially topical have been debates over the point at which government control of decision-making should give way to 'community' control over citizens' lives. Such interest manifests itself today in various ways, theoretically and in practice. Network governance, deliberative democracy, participatory democracy, citizen science and other ideas are actively debated in the literature in political science and other disciplines. In practice, community-based management of natural resources, crime prevention and emergency response procedures are widely utilized in many parts of the world. The rise in interest in market-based policy solutions (although not usually understood as being about participation) is, in fact, precisely about involvement since the solutions propose a lesser role for government and a greater role for the market and the individual. The individual may be participating as a consumer rather than as a citizen, but the degree and kind of participation have changed.

All of this is intensely political, and one should never shy away from that. A community-based wildfire protection and response management strategy, supported by state and insurance industry resources, might be viewed as a sensible operational matter. Yet, it may be reinterpreted in other ways: an expression of citizens taking control of responsibilities away from the state; a government pushing responsibilities onto local communities to cut public expenditure on professional fire agencies; or the concern of the insurance industry to reduce risk liabilities. Behind citizen participation, there often lies a range of beliefs and imperatives, and these involve different ways of negotiating and using values, resources and responsibilities: policy with an inevitable element of politics.

Governments, their agencies and other formal institutions will not always welcome participation by the wider public. Secrecy – now resurgent through security concerns and in the guise of commercial confidentiality or non-negotiable political goals – entrenched cultures of expertise and past experience may make them reluctant. This reluctance will generally increase the further up the policy hierarchy one goes – a government may support community implementation of emergency preparedness programmes, but not permit inclusion in policy formulation. While community pressure may force participation, or the options for participation may be willingly offered, either way it is crucial that if public participation is to occur, it is genuine in intent and design. False opportunities for participation, or misleading expectations of its purpose, are a waste of human resources as well as morally wrong in a democratic sense.

Clearly, public understanding of and engagement with the management, policy and institutional aspects of emergencies and disasters are both important and complex. To clarify that complexity, or at least to provide a language and structure through which it can be better understood, the following three sections explore the *who, why and how* of community participation and some relevant participatory strategies. The intent is to move beyond the mantra that 'participation is good' towards a more sophisticated and structured consideration of who might or should be included in a policy process, the purposes of that participation – that is, what 'good' is it meant to achieve – and the matching of this to different tools and options for participation.

Who? Defining 'community'

Most often, the term 'community' in many areas of policy is taken to mean a place-based subset of the population – a locality, neighbourhood or region. In emergencies and disasters, it is most often those in a specific locale or region at risk from some hazard, or else used as a general descriptor capturing the general public. This is an insufficient definition. The thing that defines a 'community' is a *commonality of interest*, which holds together, at least at particular times, a group of people and provides the impetus for shared attitudes or actions. In his classic work *Landscapes of Fear,* surely relevant to disasters, Yi-Fu Tuan (1979) explored shared threat as the basis of community. Certainly, protection against natural or human dangers was one reason for people gathering together in and creating villages and towns, but not the only reason (Boyden, 1987). Positively, a community may be based as much on shared opportunity as shared threat.

However we define community, the term conveys multiple meanings, and identification of this should inform how we think about community engagement in understanding and responding to emergencies and disasters. Table 4.1 identifies major types of common interest and the definable community attached to those in order to provide a framework for identifying different communities. Only the first is defined clearly by place, and the rest may at times have a place focus, but often do not. Table 4.1 shows the diversity of what 'community' or 'the public' comprises.

This is a simple typology, and while more detail could be developed, it suffices for the purpose of clarifying important points. First, there are clearly many 'communities' even in one small place, and these differ greatly in what they are interested in, the strength and nature of their ties to each other, the information that they may be open to, and so on. Second, individuals belong to more than one community – and generally several – which will, in multiple ways, be relevant to policy as a citizen, consumer, competitor and community member. Sensitivity to such multiple perspectives and allegiances complicate the design and implementation of participatory strategies; yet, recognition and their accommodation are imperative.

Third, commonality of interest does not imply a constant degree of agreement and collaboration – within a particular community, there may be both cooperative and competitive behaviour. For example, while the members of a real estate association may work together in the interest of the industry as a whole, individuals may be in fierce competition in the marketplace. Similarly, while the members of a local community may cooperate closely to ensure safety in the face of fire or flood threat, they may compete or even fight over other issues, or simply ignore each other.

The different communities sketched in Table 4.1 will have varying requirements and degrees of engagement with policy and management in emergencies and disasters. These will be explored further in the next section. In terms of the focus of this book – policy and institutions – they will also have very different interests in, access to and influence over the political processes that define policy directions and agendas of institutional change. Recalling terminology from Chapter 2, some may be members of the policy community, engaged in policy debates; others may be active in policy networks, exerting more influence.

This issue of influence on higher-level policy and institutional design is especially relevant in the disasters field, where it is typically the least powerful – those lacking in power, resources, political voice and influence – and who are the most severely affected. Can poor illiterate village fishermen, at risk of storm surge in cyclone seasons, be involved in high-level policy discussions, or can their knowledge and interests be fairly represented in such discussions? Conversely, should senior officials presume to understand and represent potentially affected communities? These are simplified choices, but beg the question of matching the who, why and what of community engagement and public participation in terms of selecting participatory strategies (what) that fit the community in question (who) and the purpose of participation (why).

Table 4.1 *Defining community*

Type of 'community'	Commonality of interest	Relevance to interests in disasters and emergencies (examples)
1 Place-based (spatial)	Determined by affinity with or stake in the condition of a place (neighbourhood, town or region)	Concern over the protection of local lives, livelihoods and assets at risk from natural hazards
2 Familial, kinship	Members of a located or extended family or kin network May be local to global in extent	Impacts of hazards on relatives, whether nearby or in distant locations May lobby for assistance from distant places; assistance provided to victims
3 Cultural, social, political	Communities linked by culture, ethnicity, religious belief, ideology, recreational activities, political beliefs, etc.	Risks to others in relevant community recovery programmes run through faith-based agencies, political lobbying, heritage protection groups and post-disaster activities
4 Employment, profession	Organized groups of people, often spatially dispersed, linked by profession or employment within a particular career type	Risk managers, fire-fighting professionals, floodplain managers, paramedics; individually influential at times, and as a group may advocate policy and management strategies
5 Economic, sectoral	Linked by economic interests, across or within firms and locations (e.g. car parts manufacturing, tourism industry, fishing or forestry industries)	Farmers lobby staff working on post-cyclone farm compensation, petro-chemical industry safety programmes and foresters post-fire recovery
6 Knowledge based (epistemic communities)	Communities defined by a knowledge system (e.g. an academic discipline or professional skill, such as typified by statisticians or communication managers)	Emergency management trainers, researchers, fire ecologists, floodplain hydrologists, seismologists and epidemiologists

7 Issue or topic based	Groups given identity and purpose by interest in or commitment to a substantive issue (e.g. anti-pollution campaigners, advocates for disability services, consumer protection lobbies)	Toxic chemical action networks, lobbyists focusing on flood insurance, development aid activists, land interests pushing for relaxation of development rules and commercial groups using political pressure for adoption of their disaster-relevant products
8 Emergent	May be a subset of type 7 above People who previously had little interaction can become a tightly knit group as they experience and deal with a disaster (disaster can also exacerbate pre-existing divisions)	Post-impact, the 'community' works to restore itself and may take control of its recovery Groups demanding post-disaster compensation, support and institutional change

Three examples illustrate some of the main issues:

1 *Risk awareness and sharing for wildfire community safety – community as locality.* Australian wildfire agencies are redefining their role from fire-fighting to 'community safety'. 'Community' in this context is primarily place based, but also refers to other communities (e.g. tourists) since anyone could potentially be caught in a wildfire. Community safety is seen as an explicit partnership with people at risk to jointly manage safety and property protection.

Participation varies from public information programmes aimed at the 'general public' to approaches to mobilize specific groups at risk through, for example, community fire guard, fire-wise approaches, community fire units (CFUs) and street corner meetings. These approaches are initiated and facilitated by the fire agencies, although in many cases communities will ask for support to establish a local group. One of the aims is to better prepare households and communities for wildfires, as well as to build capacity for staying and defending property during the passage of a fire. They vary in degree of participation from an interactive exchange of information to CFUs whose members are trained and equipped with basic fire-fighting gear so that they can actively protect property in their local area until fire agency crews arrive. Despite these efforts there are gaps in coverage and engagement, especially with more vulnerable groups, as well as questions of cost efficiency and resourcing.

2 *Neighbourhood groups and NGOs negotiate solutions – cultural- and issue-based*

communities. The Indian Ocean tsunami of 26 December 2004 devastated many areas, including parts of southern Thailand. Recovery and the longer-term survival and prosperity of affected areas depend on the vitality of the local economy. This means that the flow of money into and within an area affected by disaster needs to reach all of those affected. The official recovery plan explicitly recognizes the importance of money flows over simply restoring buildings, but has ignored the micro-enterprises on which many people depend, as well as the very large informal economy. Instead, it supported the more obvious economic sector of small- and medium-sized enterprises. The interests of large-scale developers were also served through, in part, enhanced access to coastal land. Many of the area's poorest people found that land they had occupied under traditional tenure was being taken from them for safety reasons to lower the exposure along the coast. However, new hotels were being constructed in this zone. Many of the more marginalized communities worked with local and international NGOs and some politicians to negotiate solutions to the land issue. They also used their local and international personal networks and religious affiliations to attract support for rebuilding and re-establishing livelihoods.

3   *Emergent community for recovery without government help.* New Orleans post-Hurricane Katrina is hardly known for community participation and recovery; but some local groups have organized themselves as 'emergent communities' (see Table 4.1). The Vietnamese population in the neighbourhood of East New Orleans was one of the poorest groups in one of the poorest cities in the US. They had limited interaction before Hurricane Katrina. After the disaster, however, local leaders emerged and the community organized to rebuild. It did so with very little help from government agencies; instead, it found itself in court opposing a contaminated waste site supported by state and local governments and located adjacent to the rebuilding community. A year after the disaster, this area has been largely rebuilt, and although one of the poorest neighbourhoods pre-Katrina appears to be thriving, restoration in most other devastated locations remains patchy and slow.

Why? Purposes and degrees of participation

Why do people believe that public participation in policy processes is a good thing and towards what end? Here we identify the broader imperatives behind moves towards more community participation in emergencies and disasters, as well as in many other areas of public policy and governance. Recognition of these broad imperatives allows understanding of the motivations behind the more specific participatory strategies discussed later:

•   disappointment with the performance of previously tried, less participatory policy and management approaches (e.g. direct expert-to-public education campaigns, regulatory policy instruments and sole state provision of emergency services), encouraging the use of policy approaches that involve a greater range of

non-state actors, such as participatory planning or community-based education or management programmes;

- to increase available resources or to redefine the problem and, thus, the range
  of strategies used (e.g. from a focus on wildfire to a focus on community safety,
  as explained above);
- alternatively, as a strategy to reduce government and/or commercial responsibility and/or expenditure by shifting responsibilities for managing emergencies
  onto communities;
- recognition of the need for local/community knowledge to be incorporated
  within emergency planning and response for logistical reasons, recognizing
  that much mitigation occurs locally, and for success needs local support if not
  active participation, and access to local knowledge. This local emphasis is even
  more important in many parts of the world where support from outside the
  disaster affected area is likely to be limited;
- mistrust of government and the institutions of the state to represent community values and preferences, whether based on actual experience or a generic
  political position;
- a range of other agendas, including harnessing public pressure to promote
  commercial and political ends (e.g. high-profile technologies for fire-fighting
  and hurricane risk reduction);
- general political belief in participatory democracy and the fundamental value
  of participation, rather than representative democracy or centralized control;
  this is the only case where public participation is an end in itself – in the points
  above, it is a means to some other end.

These different imperatives have at their basis contrasting logic and beliefs about
how society should be governed, and the roles and responsibilities of the citizen
and the state. There is a broad split between participation that is demanded from
the 'bottom up' (community insistence) and participation that is pushed from
the 'top down' (by government); but, commonly, a mixture of the two will be
evident. Not recognizing the existence of multiple contrasting understandings of
participation in a given situation may lead to misunderstanding and mistrust, and
to hidden assumptions and tensions. Alternatively, made visible and discussed, such
diversity in motive could provide positive opportunities for mutual understanding
and cooperation to achieve multiple ends. The community desiring control and
the government desiring efficiencies in programme delivery may be in conflict
or collaboration, depending on the degree of mutual understanding of these two
agendas. Commercial imperatives are increasingly likely to complicate this picture
as companies lobby for endorsement and purchase of their emergency management
products and services.

Beneath these general imperatives there are more specific purposes of participation, and some are identified in Table 4.2.

As with the broad imperatives behind participation, these more specific purposes
are quite different, although not necessarily always in conflict. However, the potential for misunderstanding and conflict – and for participation approaches that are
inefficient or ineffective – is increased in situations where different purposes are

Table 4.2 *Main purposes of public participation*

Purpose	Explanation
1 Gain participation in social debates	Encourage debate about broader social values and goals, and the construction and understanding of social and policy problems, such as general approaches to responsibilities regarding disasters and emergencies
2 Inform and legitimate policy formulation	Inform and define policy problems, formulate policy or develop policy principles that have widespread understanding and acceptance
3 Ensure transparency and accountability	Ensure transparency and accountability in the policy process in order to enhance trust in policy and institutions, or efficiency in the use of resources
4 Enforcement	Ensure enforcement of, and compliance with, policy, whether through alerting authorities, input into commissions of inquiry or legal action in the courts
5 Access information, including monitoring	Incorporate expertise or information within the policy process, such as local knowledge and experience regarding risk, hazard events, community attitudes and preparedness
6 Enable policy monitoring and learning	Monitor and evaluate policy and management interventions using community resources and expertise, with feedback to problem definition and policy choice
7 Aid policy and programme implementation	Implement or aid implementation of policy instruments or policy programmes through community (or parts of community) collaboration
8 Engage in on-ground management	Engage in operational emergency management: preparedness, response and recovery
9 Share the risk	Share the responsibilities and costs associated with identified risks between government and the communities at risk

not recognized by the actors involved. The various 'communities' identified in Table 4.1 will see participation as fulfilling different purposes. An epistemic community (e.g. fire ecologists) may view a community monitoring programme as a means of generating vegetation recovery data, the local community as part of its preparedness for fire events, and an environmental action network as an input into endangered species protection measures. Commonly, an individual or organization will have more than one reason and purpose to demand or offer greater participation.

The contrasting purposes of participation relate to different parts of the policy process (see Figure 3.2 in Chapter 3) and locations in the institutional and organizational landscape (see Table 2.1 in Chapter 2). In stages 1 and 2 (problem framing and strategic policy choice) of the policy framework, participation focuses on purposes 1, 2 and 6 above (social debate over general goals, deciding policy directions and informing the redefinition of policy problems). In stage 3, purposes such as 5, 7 and 8 would be most relevant. In stage 4 (policy monitoring and learning), the obvious purpose is policy monitoring (point 6 in Table 4.2). These suggest very different approaches to community engagement and public participation, as discussed below.

In the case of participation and institutional location (see Table 2.1), the public may have influence at the highest level, via punishing or rewarding a government for their performance in handling disasters through the ballot box. At a place-based level, local government may be similarly influenced by the electorate or a district office of a government emergency service agency may seek involvement of the community in monitoring or management, or be lobbied by residents for better services. In the aftermath of a disaster, superior courts may hear cases against authorities, or residents' groups, industry associations and others may give evidence to coronial inquests or commissions of inquiry.

Different purposes imply a range of degrees of relationship between citizens and the state, and between citizens and agencies of the state. To achieve the purpose of informing social and policy goals, and strategic policy choice, some entry of non-state actors into policy networks is implicit. In contrast, engagement by local residents in operational management and monitoring typically involves a formalized, yet more distant, relationship – larger policy decisions are made within government, but communities are involved in implementation. The trend to community risk management (see Chapter 1) has largely involved such operational relationships, rather than significant changes in who has influence over strategic policy choice and related discussions within powerful policy networks.

Degrees of participation

What is the appropriate degree of participation that is desirable or necessary in a particular set of circumstances? Arnstein's (1969) classic 'ladder of participation' comprised eight 'rungs', with the lowest, manipulation and therapy, involving little citizen or public power, then moving through informing, consulting, placating and partnership, up to the higher levels of delegated power and citizen control. Advocates of participatory democracy tend to view more participation as better, whereas those who believe in the effectiveness of strong government, or who doubt the ability of communities and citizens to make informed judgements and undertake important tasks, may exhibit an overall preference for less participation. A similar preference comes from those who argue that we have governments and agencies to take responsibility for decisions and actions on behalf of citizens, not to simply pass on such responsibilities. Yet, if we accept a wide range of 'communities' and of purposes for participation (above), and an equally wide range of participatory processes and tools, then the real question becomes: is the degree of participation appropriate to the issue at hand and to the needs and values of those involved?

Individuals and groups who may fall into a particular category of 'community' will have varying needs, desires and tolerances with respect to participation.
Some members of a local community may seek to be deeply engaged in developing
emergency policy and procedures; others are satisfied simply with knowing what is
happening; others again may have no time for either. Participation is usually voluntary, and volunteer capacity is a scarce resource to be used wisely and efficiently.
Denial of a problem and refusal to engage in, for example, hazard minimization,
is a personal choice. Forced participation equals command and control, but may
be justified if the safety of others is threatened or if there is a risk of large public
costs. The provision of different degrees of participation, of opportunities to climb
up and down the 'ladder', and, indeed, to jump on and off the ladder, are necessary
considerations in the design of participatory strategies. Arnstein's (1969) classification concerns degrees and types of *active and intentional* participation. However,
even if unaware of the fact, non-participating individuals participate by sharing the
risk passively with insurers and government by virtue of simply being at risk.

Participation not only has a cost in terms of community time and effort, but
must be weighed against family life, employment and other community activities. Participatory policy approaches that are inclusive of more actors in institutional systems, may produce better outcomes; but they also demand time, financial
resources, and human skills and effort by all concerned. A public-sector agency
rarely replaces existing functions with a participatory approach, but rather adds
participation to an existing suite of policy tasks and administrative processes.
For example, by redefining its business from fire-fighting to community safety,
a fire agency will need to engage with those at risk while retaining and, perhaps,
enhancing its traditional capabilities. In an era of public-sector downsizing, this
can create tensions and, moreover, requires quite different skills from traditional
approaches to public policy and, thus, perhaps necessitates specific personnel. Such
costs should not be ignored since poorly executed participatory processes will not
only produce poor policy outcomes, but may also erode trust and willingness to
engage in further activities.

In some areas of public policy, there are limits to participation that should be
recognized and openly discussed, and the field of emergencies and disasters is a
particular case. The costs of non-participation may involve a reasoned or ignorant
discounting of risk to one's self; but non-participation may also place others at risk.
This begs intervention by society, usually represented by an agency of the state such
as an emergency services authority. In times of imminent event onset, the real time
imperatives of an emergency allow limited room only for active participation to be
negotiated, and if roles and responses are not well defined, in practice (and, later,
defendable in law), then confusion and worse are likely.

Many of the key themes presented at the end of Chapter 1 reinforce the importance of closely considering both the key role of participation in increasing the
resilience of communities and in choosing strategies to encourage and allow it. The
whole-of-society character of emergencies and disasters requires whole-of-society
engagement in problem framing and strategic policy choice. The inevitability of
residual uncertainty suggests that roles should be defined for handling the possibility of thresholds and surprise, and the existence of multiple aims and values

demands engagement in policy by those who hold those values. The marginalized situation of those most often affected by disasters demands strategies that open up policy discussions and institutions to the views and values of those people who are very often least engaged in formal and traditional processes of policy and governance.

This last point – participation by the marginalized – presents an especially difficult challenge when we stretch the emergency policy domain to enhancing the resilience of local communities and economies pre- and post-event, rather than simply emphasizing preparedness, response and recovery. Participation by communities in land-use planning, diversification of economic livelihoods, maintenance of appropriate infrastructure for transport and communications, local health programmes, risk sharing and shifting via insurance, politics and media, and so on – these greatly extend the scope of community engagement in disaster policy in terms of the agencies and portfolios of government involved, individuals and organizations relevant, time and skills required, and specific approaches employed. We now turn to the latter.

How? Options for community engagement

The practical options available to allow, encourage or ensure public participation and community engagement are numerous. Here, we survey and comment on the main options. To link participatory strategies and methods more explicitly to the outcomes desired and their most appropriate context, this section groups them (with some overlap) to the *purposes of participation* identified in Table 4.2. The detailed design of processes across widely different situations is not the topic here; rather, it is to scope the range of options and general differences in their appropriate uses.

Purpose 1: Social debate and problem framing. Wider involvement in broad social and policy debate about disasters and emergencies is desirable to:

- involve the necessary multiple perspectives and values in these debates;
- increase the likelihood of acceptance of ensuing problem definitions and policy directions; and
- help move emergency management concerns into the political mainstream.

Options for the policy network and others to increase such participation include:

- seeking to have emergency policy placed on the ongoing political agenda, given that it is very often absent except immediately post-event; political parties and senior government figures are the most obvious target, whether directly or through the media;
- parliamentary inquiries or similar processes, with calls for public input and a public reporting process;
- reframing emergency management to link with existing major political concerns, such as climate change or social and economic development goals.

Purpose 2: Strategic policy choice and policy formulation. This is perhaps the largest gap in current practice, involving a move far beyond governments communicating the importance of disasters and seeking implementation by communities of policy and procedures towards engagement of the public or their representatives in discussing the broad directions of emergency policy. Options for enabling such engagement include:

- various publicly visible and accessible inquiry processes focusing on overarching aspects of disasters (e.g. community resilience, policy styles and problem framing);
- broadened community membership of processes within the policy system to allow further development of disaster policy as a whole-of-society policy domain through inclusion of representatives of, for example, community development, natural resource management, infrastructure and utilities, economic policy, primary industry, micro-enterprises, public health and education, alongside the more traditional emergency-oriented interests;
- increased connection across public agencies, reflecting sectors as per the above point, in the form of task forces, interdepartmental committees or conferences, or joint implementation teams;
- greater attention to risks and emergencies in existing processes that allow community input into relevant decision-making, such as land-use planning systems and building standards design.

Purpose 3: Transparency and accountability. Emergency management is often tested in public with immediate, if not real-time, feedback during (and often for long after) a major disaster. Political and media scrutiny of those involved may be intense, interfering and unforgiving. On the other hand, fire and emergency services are among the most trusted and respected of public services, and criticism may be limited for that reason. In these important respects, emergency management differs from other sectors in its accountability and transparency. Processes to achieve transparency and accountability include:

- intense media scrutiny, which is difficult to deflect during and immediately after a disaster, making it hard to avoid accountability (however, this may focus on issues beyond the control of emergency managers, and strategic questions may be less visible and escape public examination);
- regular and visible reviews of policy efficacy through auditor investigations, inquiries, parliamentary committee inquiries, etc.;
- normal accountability mechanisms of public administration, including freedom of information provisions, publicly available annual reports, limits to commercial in confidence provisions, etc.;
- community and interest group representation on key policy formulation and review bodies, allowing for scrutiny and communication by a wider range of interests;
- full use of the feedback mechanisms that are integral to risk management processes;

- an active and engaged research community.

Purpose 4: Enforcement and compliance. A high level of transparency and accountability should help to ensure compliance and may assist with enforcement. A clearly set out policy with a sound evidence base also helps by minimizing uncertainty and any suggestion that the approach is arbitrary. Options include:

- appropriate avenues for legal recourse and review of expenditure, planning and performance, with sufficient rules of standing to allow genuine (but not vexatious) actions through the courts;
- linkages between community-based monitoring and management activities and higher-level policy processes and institutional locations of authority, allowing community reporting of performance;
- inclusion of *local* government (with necessary resources) in policy and management programmes as the most directly accessible of democratically legitimate levels of government, responsible for control of many zoning, building, etc. functions;
- quality information systems that make performance reporting possible and available to relevant interests;
- processes for negotiating between competing interests that undermine compliance.

Purpose 5: Information inputs to policy. This is often a major gap, with policy lacking information input from those whom it will most affect. Researchers and research results are often directly connected with community and other stakeholders, and are in a position to pass this information on to emergency managers and policy-makers, provided appropriate mechanisms exist. Approaches include:

- surveys, polls, focus groups and other data-gathering mechanisms, connected to policy formulation and implementation processes;
- participatory research programmes, connecting research to affected communities and to community-based management programmes;
- active designing-in of experimentation and evaluation to policy and management interventions in order to ensure routine data capture and lesson drawing;
- informal ways of being alerted to useful information (since formal links with all relevant information sources are probably impossible, in part, because all needs cannot be predicted); these may include participation in seminars run by research groups and scanning of a wide range of current research publications.

Purpose 6: Policy learning. Each disaster, near miss, rehearsal and risk analysis offers opportunities for learning and improvement. There is much rhetoric on this topic; but real learning involving significant change is often very slow in practice. Learning at the level of operational detail is much simpler than that requiring institutional change. Unfortunately, opportunities for learning and change can become politically charged blaming exercises, with the result that shifting blame becomes the primary objective rather than learning. Options to help ensure participatory learning include:

- expanded representation of committees, advisory bodies, etc., according to above for strategic policy choice;
- post-event review and evaluation processes of inquiry, mandated to glean lessons for broader policy and management aspects as opposed to event-specific or liability-focused inquiries (discussed further in Chapter 8);
- independent reviews of major post-event inquiries to ensure that the process has not been captured by special interests to the exclusion of the interests of those at risk;
- development of whole-of-sector communication pathways and information and human resources, including educational and training pathways to enhance capacities and knowledge in policy, as well as in operational management;
- use of negotiation processes to encourage cooperation across government and interest groups;
- taking advantage of crises anywhere, as well as anniversaries, to involve community members directly in promoting awareness and appropriate actions.

Purpose 7: Policy and programme implementation. At this level, formal community participation is too often absent; yet, this is the level that sets the context for operational emergency management where people have no option but involvement simply through being at risk. We argue that community or, rather, stakeholder input and involvement can be valuable and help to deliver the desired outcomes, and in many circumstances it may be essential to implementation. In addition to the people at risk, infrastructure and utility providers, often from the private sector, may be key players. Important aspects of implementation are often under the control of groups who would normally be seen as existing outside emergency management: utility provision and regulatory processes are among the more obvious of these. Less obvious may be the role of markets for certain goods and services, and the myriad of factors in community resilience, including income security and health services. A strong trend is towards an expanding number of organizations seeing themselves as having an emergency management role, including:

- regional coordination of different emergency services, with community representatives on committees and boards;
- local business, whose support (especially local development interests) will often be crucial to successful implementation;
- involvement of utility providers (water, energy, etc.) in policy processes and implementation;
- presentations to, or membership of, strategic planning committees by those at risk;
- policy-relevant committees with broad membership – most easily achieved through advisory rather than decision-making bodies.

Purpose 8: Operational emergency management. As mentioned earlier, people, organizations and commerce cannot avoid being involved informally at this level – when disaster strikes their locations, they will participate (although this may not apply to institutionalized populations or to those completely dependent on carers).

Informal involvement can take many forms. Formal involvement possibilities range from emergency managers seeking advice from people at risk, through to explicitly sharing the risk and handing operations over to local people:

- Formal community-based management processes, such as neighbourhood fire groups, flood-warning monitoring programmes and lifeline support programmes that share the risk explicitly. In some cases, such groups may assume full operational responsibility; but more often they play important component roles (e.g. by securing themselves, their livelihoods and properties).
- Informal, unplanned local assistance during an emergency; dealing with 'spontaneous volunteers', people who simply turn up wanting to help at the disaster scene but without training or equipment, is often an issue for emergency managers and is frequently viewed as a problem. The problem can be exacerbated: often, many people are there to look rather than to help. This is part of the well-established problem of convergence in disasters. Nevertheless, in major disasters, especially if they involve extensive areas, the first responders will usually be local people, untrained and informally organized at best.
- Participation by commerce through risk sharing, formally by offering insurance, and less formally though providing aid and credit during and after the immediate impact. Commerce also typically participates formally or informally by providing resources and expertise, and by allowing emergency service volunteers to take time off work. In many countries organized volunteers are the mainstay of emergency management operations, and businesses far from the location of the emergency may find that they bear significant costs as staff are called to emergency operations.
- During and after immediate impact, risk-sharing by both the affected community and commerce may have an international dimension. This often involves global commerce by insurers spreading their risk internationally through reinsurance, and international companies supporting the affected part of the company. For events that receive significant publicity, people rich and poor everywhere donate aid for the affected areas. The fact that such aid – including operational support – may be inappropriate or even counter-productive is the subject of a large literature, and guidelines on disaster aid should always be consulted (see, for example, www.reliefweb.int under *Resources*). There are also situations where those affected by disaster appear to be largely ignored by their own governments or the international community (see Médecins sans Frontières, www.msf. org). In major and minor events, people mobilize their personal networks and send and receive resources across the world to their friends, relatives and home towns. In many areas of the world, receipt of such funds or remittances is an important source of day-to-day income, and helps to buffer the recipients from local emergencies.

Across all of the above, there is an implied hierarchy of relevance within the policy system. The various purposes, and the approaches that match to them, engage with broader or more specific processes and organizational locations. Recalling Table 2.1, some connect with the institutional system through parliament, some through public-sector agencies, some through non-state actors, some through commercial markets, and others through the courts.

The broad options listed above are used in the emergencies and disasters field, some more than others. This situation is not stable for several reasons. The number of groups that see themselves as part of emergency management is increasing, fuelled by massive growth of the security sector and recognition of business vulnerability to emergencies. It also appears that in much of the world, people's expectations of emergency management are increasing. Combining these two macro trends in participation and expectations suggests that improved processes are needed to manage expectations and to negotiate between the different priorities of the growing range of stakeholders. Community risk management approaches may help with this.

Deliberative designs

A distinct suite of participatory options, increasingly advocated (although far less often formally incorporated within policy processes), are captured under the term deliberative designs: operational methods drawn from the theoretical ideal of deliberative democracy (e.g. Dryzek, 2000; Munton, 2002). These are structured methods, utilizing careful selection of participants as representatives of society to inform either problem framing or policy design. This represents a departure from the typical bases of participation: voluntary community participation in processes created by public agencies; representation or advocacy through normal political processes, aimed at influencing public policy, which includes pressure through the media; and the activities of organized interest groups. It has major implications for existing interest groups, whose status and roles are recast, and for public agencies, who may end up sponsoring a process that defines problems or responses not in keeping with its own beliefs or priorities.

Deliberative designs include a range of methods, suited to different purposes. Citizens' juries, for example, entail a selected representative group of lay citizens considering an issue over a number of days, gaining and judging information inputs and expert witnesses before arriving at conclusions. Consensus conferences and deliberative polls are larger-scale approaches based on a similar logic. An array of methods in the area of multi-criteria analysis (MCA) may be used to consider multiple values and goals, and some MCA methods are inclusive in design, where community representatives use the structure and rigour of MCA to guide and direct their own problem- and response-framing discussions. A variety of integrated assessment methods also exist that are relevant to emergency policy and planning. This area is large and rapidly evolving, with many proposed approaches and an increasing variety of applications, although generally of weak status within formal policy processes.

Approaches such as these are suited to different purposes and contexts. For example, consensus conferences are suited to larger policy questions, whereas integrated assessment or MCA are suited to more defined and place-specific issues. None, however, are cheap or necessarily quick ways of including community perspectives and, thus, should be used sparingly, in a strategic manner and only when the outcomes are to be taken seriously.

Inclusion as exclusion

An important aspect of choosing a participatory strategy is the exclusion of some people or issues that may be inherent in decisions to include others – the decision of who, why and how will often entail an implicit judgement that other communities, purposes and options are excluded. The choice of approach or structure will also define the issues to be dealt with and, therefore, also those issues not on the agenda, and the forms of information input that will and will not be used. Such limitation may be appropriate and justified on the basis of careful analysis; but it may be done unthinkingly (perhaps even very deliberately). For example, a decision to run a participatory planning process at a regional rather than local district scale may include those with regional interests, but exclude some whose interests are specific to one locale or who lack the resources to engage at a wider geographical scale. Similarly, the choice of communication media may exclude those who do not or cannot access that media (e.g. the internet). Inadvertent exclusion by government will most likely occur at local scales or with specific programmes, whereas intentional exclusion is more likely at higher levels of policy formulation. However, given wider participation in the problem framing and strategic choice elements of the policy process (see Figure 3.2), inadvertent exclusion of people and interests becomes less likely.

A related and crucial consideration in participatory approaches is that of *representation*. Local community representatives may or may not faithfully represent the diversity of values and interests in the local population. Industry organizations may be biased, knowingly or not, towards only part of the sector (e.g. many smaller or fewer larger firms). The interests of very small or micro-firms and those of the informal economic sector are often under-represented or excluded, even though they account for the bulk of local employment. Expert members of teams running participatory modelling exercises may have disciplinary, methodological or personal preferences that influence who becomes involved, the data gathered and used, and the techniques employed. The use of deliberative techniques involves a recasting of actors, with selected members of the general community being assigned a very different role than usual, and deeply engaged members of expert or interest organizations shifted from advocates to interrogated witnesses. There are no neat answers to the issue of representation other than to recognize it and to carefully assess the communities of interest and the purpose of participation, and to match this consideration with the choice of approach.

Principles for participation

Considerations such as those discussed so far in this chapter invite a distillation of principles to guide formal participatory approaches to policy and institutions in the context of emergencies and disasters. A number of these have been identified in this chapter already, and the following brings these together for clarity:

- If more participatory policy processes are used, then the *intent and process should be clear* to all involved in terms of their regard for community perspectives and openness to those perspectives having influence.

- Participation should be supported by *sufficient resources*, including information, organizational capacity, skills and finance.
- Participation should be enabled for an *adequate time* period for the purpose, noting that this will vary significantly across problems.
- The time scale of participatory approaches for enhancing *community resilience* should essentially be open ended.
- Public participation and community engagement should be *efficient*. Engagement is almost always voluntary and even though the benefits to communities may be significant, the scarcity of the resource of volunteerism instructs that processes should be efficient in order to avoid wasted time and effort, and to allow for wider participation.
- Those relevant to the problem should be included, demanding a reasonably *fine-scale understanding of the 'community'*, and multiple participatory strategies are necessary in order to include all parts of the community.
- There should be sensitivity to the potential for a specific participatory design to *exclude* some people or interests, even unwittingly. Exclusion always has the potential to backfire on the organizers, especially given the inherent unpredictability of the emergency field.
- Attention should be paid to the inclusion of *marginalized or less powerful* individuals and groups, who are often the worst affected by disaster and have the least capacity for recovery.
- Participating individuals and groups should be made aware of the *limits of knowledge and uncertainties* surrounding the issues.
- All involved should be cognizant of the view that participation in emergency management is ideally about *collaboration* (doing with) rather than direction (doing to).
- Strategies, methods and processes for participation should be selected from a *wide set of options*, suited to different but equally valid *purposes*.
- Given that participation seeks to increase understanding and coordination in human societies, *communication and information* are an essential component of participatory policy strategies and are two-way processes. Both those at risk and agencies require this understanding.

Policy processes that are consistent with these principles are by no means easier; in fact, they are more complicated and difficult. Yet, if the outcomes and defensibility of policy with wider inputs and ownership are likely to be better, as is widely argued, then engaging with, rather than ignoring, this complexity and difficulty will produce better processes and outcomes. To finish this chapter, we now turn to an expansion of the final principle: communication.

Communication: The lifeblood of participation

The engagement of a wider proportion of the population in emergencies and disaster policy places significant demands on capacities to generate, transfer and utilize information: in short, communication. The most widely accepted communication imperative regarding disasters is the transfer of appropriate information concerning the nature of risks faced, what to do in the case of an event, and post-event assistance and recovery strategies and resources. The art and craft of such communication is core business to the emergency management sector, and is the subject of a large theoretical and practical literature on risk communication (see, for example, articles in the journal *Risk Analysis,* and many websites accessible via links at www.colorado.edu/hazards; see also Twigg, 2004). Here, the focus on the policy and institutional aspects of disasters invites a different perspective – on communication pathways to enhance public participation, especially in strategic policy choice, and the institutional settings conducive to enhancing such participation.

Policy directions arise from the sharing of information and perspectives, and discussing this with policy networks and communities. Greater participation of a broader range of perspectives in disaster policy – either the public directly or their representatives – enlarges the policy community, and demands a transformation of information types and pathways. New actors will inevitably require new communication forms and bring new forms of information with them into the policy process, including local empirical knowledge. Many of the participatory approaches surveyed above, such as deliberative methods and inclusion of cross-sectoral representatives within existing policy forums, serve to bring new perspectives into policy discourses. Two important considerations arise here: the role of information in policy processes and the different modes of communication required in more participatory policy processes (these issues are explored further in Chapter 7).

On the first of these, the role of information in policy processes, a common assumption must be unseated. Too often, it is assumed that information has or should have a linear cause–effect relationship to policy – the assumption of rational utilization, where information produces a rational response in the form of policy change. In fact, rational utilization of information is rare or, at least, very hard to establish. As an arena of multiple and contested values, agendas, compromise and political decisions based on ideology, expediency and pragmatism, policy does not often wait – or simply cannot afford to wait – for the best possible information on which to base decisions. Rather, a satisfactory or tolerable level of information is often the most that is available.

A single form or source of information is rarely involved, but rather a mix of political judgement, public attitudes, expert reports and so on. In such a decision-making environment, information is utilized in less than rational ways, and understandably so. We can consider a number of forms of information utilization, summarized as follows (from Hezri, 2004, drawing on an extensive empirical and theoretical literature in knowledge utilization):

- *instrumental use*, where information directly and demonstrably influences a policy or management decision;
- *conceptual use*, where information percolates into the understanding of the recipients, influencing their understanding of problems and of cause and effect;
- *political and symbolic use*, where information is used for tactical or strategic reasons in the interests of the individual or group.

Much is made of the rapidly evolving world of contemporary information and communication technology. We are not concerned here with communication during a crisis other than the issue of planning for such circumstances. New modes of communication are often seen as a panacea, with the use of websites often viewed as solving communication problems. Certainly, the internet has made it easy to have documents and other material readily available at low cost and to have interactive discussion groups and bulletin boards – in short, to exchange views and ideas. Nevertheless, achieving 'communication' as an interactive engagement between people remains challenging.

Communication research has been dominated by commercial and political questions of how to persuade people at a distance and, from a distance, how to make the communication experience more personal and therefore persuasive. Modern communication technologies may have reduced the credibility gap between face-to-face encounters and communication at a distance. However, a reasonable level of consensus exists to the effect that face-to-face encounters remain the preferred way of communicating, where results depend on mutual understanding, negotiation and persuasion – trust remains a key factor whether in an interagency situation or working with communities (see Irwin, 1995).

The strong trend towards evidence-based policy and practice in many areas, including emergency management – albeit within the context set out above of competing interests and agendas – demands an appropriate information base: appropriate in the sense that it provides usable material for emergency management. It may be unfortunate; but information in scientific journals and other specialized fora that may be directly relevant to policy development is often not consulted and incorporated within policy. An exception would be scientific information on many natural hazards. However, there are numerous examples where such information has been suppressed or sidelined: this has happened to flood-related information around the world, and some governments have actively sidelined debate on climate change and variability. Nevertheless, policy drawing on firm evidence abounds (e.g. the Australian wildfire and London smog cases set out in Chapter 1). Flood, earthquake and hurricane wind-related regulations are based on science globally, as are regulations for industrial and transportation hazards, although frequently there are questions about implementation (see Chapter 6). Local knowledge, derived from consultation and engagement with communities at risk, is often key to emergency management success or failure, especially in implementation. It is not found in the world of science.

Emergency management relies on a number of types of information for policy development and implementation – primarily, information on hazards, whether physical, technological or of some other source; on the assets, including people and activities, at risk; and on local emergency management-relevant capacities (both tangible, such as infrastructure, and intangible, such as people's mental preparedness). Important but less obvious information is found in local knowledge and concerns local procedures and capacities for implementing risk-related regulations and policy, the realities of the institutional legal and political contexts, and local customs and habits that may affect emergency management thinking and practice. Development and economic status and trends may also be relevant. This material is used as the basis for land-use planning, building codes, to identify vulnerabilities from which to develop policies for enhancing resilience, for risk management, and to support emergency preparedness and planning.

If we consider the question of 'who needs to know what?' we can match these different forms of information with appropriate 'communities'.

Communication challenges

There are several persistent communication challenges facing emergency management, apart from those posed by new media and its differential uptake across demographic groups. A fundamental difficulty is that much information that should be drawn on is not generally available in a form that makes it useful for emergency planning. Development and local system testing with community participation remains the most reliable approach for emergency communications.

Communicating across government agencies has long been a complicated challenge with distinct disciplines, worldviews, politics and missions. An engineering agency with flood-related responsibility might have trouble dealing with emergency managers, or with planners who have their social and commercial orientations. Inter-agency committees have many names, including task forces and working groups; but their function is similar: to bring often disparate groups together to focus on a common aim. While many exist more on paper than in action, in some jurisdictions they are seen as fundamental to making emergency management work.

Other key issues facing communication include the following:

- Dialogue is a fundamental issue in achieving communication in the full sense of two-way interaction between all parties, as opposed to the easy but far less useful monologue or advertising approach. The latter is less useful since we do not know if the message has been heard, much less understood or accepted.
- Information overload: in disaster planning, much will appear potentially relevant, especially as additional stakeholders become involved. The amount may appear overwhelming, and a substantial amount of knowledge will not be in a form that makes it easy to use.
- Disparate constructions of uncertainty and complexity are often one of the larger gaps between officials, scientists and those at risk, with the latter emphasizing trust and the potential impact on themselves. Officials and scientists focus on the abstract of numerical probabilities and on the impersonal aspects of impact. Sometimes this is reversed, however: the cases of suppressing climate change and floodplain information have been mentioned earlier, whereas Y2K (the millennium bug) and terrorism are examples where officials have emphasized emotion over data as one approach to uncertainty.
- Indifference and fatalism: in some remote areas and poorer countries, the arrival of officials to discuss emergency management will elicit great excitement among those at risk. However, often even being noticed by a significant proportion of those at risk can be challenging until an event occurs. The fact that people have many day-to-day priorities and concerns, sometimes about their very survival,

is well documented, resulting in disaster prevention being well down the list of priorities. Some groups – for reasons of powerlessness, religious belief or belief that responsibility lies elsewhere, such as with government – appear uninterested in disaster issues.

- Political sensitivities are important in all areas of public policy. While they may limit what can be done at any one time, circumstances can change and sensitivities will follow. Often simply repackaging the message will remove the political problem.
- Commercial-in-confidence and privatization: increasingly, aspects of emergency service work (e.g. technological services, specialist equipment and services, and in some areas the entire service, such as ambulance services in parts of the US) are in the hands of commercial organizations. One issue here is that information may be seen as a commercial commodity and, therefore, protected. In addition, commerce is naturally driven by making money rather than necessarily a cost-effective or adequate approach to service delivery.
- There is a strong trend to privilege security against terrorism and crime over other hazards, with the accompanying difficulty that information in these areas, particularly counter-terrorism, is considered secret for national security reasons.

These last two (and sometimes last three) points have the effect of making information on disaster management secret or, at least, very difficult to obtain for those at risk and even for those expected to plan for disaster.

Short societal attention spans and rapid amnesia are the bane of disaster victims and many emergency managers, and a boon for those avoiding responsibility. There is a frequent political desire to look forward rather than backwards at a disaster. In this they may be reflecting the notorious mass media tendency to move quickly to 'new' news. As a result, victims often feel abandoned despite the promises made in the glare of the international media spotlight. In this there is an awkward balance to be negotiated between avoiding expensive blaming exercises and some visibility so that the longer-term recovery needs of those affected are not ignored. Many enquiries done in the name of learning lead to heightened caution, with insignificant changes as far as those at risk are concerned.

Conclusion

In emergency management the meaning of 'community' is expanding rapidly as an increasing number and range of groups realize that emergency management is part of their remit. We acknowledge that the term 'community' has many valid definitions and that emergency management policy needs to take account of these. Expanding involvement away from a select group of specialists towards engagement with many potential stakeholders is part of achieving broad-based ownership and mainstreaming emergency management policy.

More players, each with their own agendas and priorities, almost inevitably lead to more complex patterns of participation, with greater demands on emergency managers. Participation can come in many formal and informal forms. The use of markets may involve both forms. While this involves greater opportunities for public input into policy, it also increases demands for time, skills and resources to make such participation effective.

Participation involves communication, and the essence of communication is establishing dialogue or engagement. It is not simply a one-way transfer of information, which is unlikely to be successful anyway without some degree of engagement. Policy requires processes that engage with the broad range of 'communities' and stakeholders both for policy development and implementation and, in many cases, to assist with operational measures.

Framing the Problem: Identifying and Analysing Risk

To create effective policy we need to be clear about what problem or issues the policy is intended to address. Even an apparently straightforward risk will invite many ways of thinking about the problem. Fundamental differences and gaps in risk comprehension have long been documented across communities at risk, the broader public, scientists analysing the risk, and politicians and emergency managers who have to find workable solutions. Underlying these different perspectives will be distinct ways of framing the problem. While all might agree that there is a problem (e.g. a flood threat) and even on the symptoms, there is likely to be conflict over the causes and on what to do. To some extent, and sometimes to a large extent, this conflict will emerge from the way in which the problem is framed. The simple question: 'What is the problem?' will elicit a range of views that must be negotiated as policy is developed drawing on the approaches set out in Chapters 4 and 6.

Here we clarify concepts and provide an overview of proximate and underlying causes, problem definition (generally and through risk assessment), social, environmental and economic costs estimation, and institutional implications.

Problem framing

How we define and frame problems will circumscribe our search for solutions. Many specific ways of framing problems will constrain the search for solutions and may lead to important issues being ignored – for example, by focusing on what we know well or find easy to measure. As a result, it is useful to examine risk using multiple framings. Recognizing and applying different perspectives will highlight where important issues may lie and who stands to lose from different policies. But this may be difficult to do because some of the drivers of problem framing are fundamental to society and it can be difficult to step outside dominant institutional or disciplinary ways of thinking. Of course, this raises the issue as to who frames problems and why. Any stakeholder can frame or reframe the problem; but some are more influential. The media are powerful problem framers in most policy arenas; they may lead or often follow framing by political leaders, commerce may frame problems to their advantage, and so on. Framing can occur at a number of levels from the generic to policy dealing with a single hazard. Here we touch on both levels.

Some reasons for rethinking policy problems in emergency management include:

- a desire to put emergency management into the policy mainstream, not as a marginal activity;
- dealing with causes rather than symptoms, leading to the need for strategic thinking;
- shifting responsibility or blame (e.g. institutional issues *versus* natural hazard agents, or human error *versus* malevolence);
- the need for appropriate institutional structures to deliver long-term solutions;
- sharing ownership of the problem with those at risk and working to reduce vulnerability through education and other programmes.

Drivers for different ways of framing problems include:

- disciplinary perspectives and worldviews (see below);
- legal requirements and the need to avoid liability and legal risk;
- political considerations, where disasters create political risk, cause political opportunities that favour specific groups or result in the blaming of identifiable groups or nature;
- government legitimacy, where in addition to the politics of blame and generosity, disasters and disaster management provide opportunities for politicians to show their power, control and leadership;
- economic and commercial imperatives, when disaster management may be seen as too expensive and conflicting with local economic goals; alternatively, commercial interest may see advantages in promoting concern, such as Y2K (the millennium computer bug), the security industry or sensationalist media;
- fear and perceptions that disaster is likely to stigmatize an area; alternatively, there may be fear of the mitigation effort, such as prescribed burning to reduce wildfire risk, provision of flood-related information with implications for property prices, or circulation of emergency plans to those living near hazardous industrial or storage sites;
- a common view that the availability of insurance is an important factor in risk-taking, discounting the need for other actions.

If we consider strategies for emergency management we can see that they might change depending on how the problem is defined. Take the example of flooding:

- *The problem is the hazard (the physical phenomenon).* With floodwater, the objective might be to manage the water, and the approach would logically be flood walls and other engineering works. Traditionally, The Netherlands epitomizes this approach, and New Orleans shows its limits. Applying the same objective, another approach, now finding favour with planning authorities, might be to hold water in catchments where it falls, or to retain it in natural or artificial features – which, although not intended for floodwater control, can be turned to that function. These different approaches to the same objective highlight the varying approaches between engineering agencies, land management agencies and planners.

- *The problem is one of exposure to the hazard.* The objective would be to reduce exposure of people and activities to floodwater, achieved through planning regulations that prohibit development in flood-prone areas. But this is often difficult in areas with strong development pressure, areas that are often likely to also be prone to flooding (e.g. near rivers or the sea) or where unplanned informal settlements are the only places for people to establish dwellings. There are many options for defining flood prone land. Similarly, planners might limit development of coastal locations because of storm surge hazard, or put in place exclusion zones around hazardous industries and storage sites.

- *The problem is that some communities are especially vulnerable to flooding, and the objective will be to reduce that.* The problem may be related to exposure, as above, but may also be that flooding affects the community's livelihoods – so the emphasis could be on local economic security. Perhaps flooding would impact on health, so the policy could target health and housing quality, and so on. The vulnerability issue can be framed in many ways, including culturally, historically and politically. In any case, the focus is on reducing the consequences of flooding on the people affected. Many people in poorer areas prefer this type of approach as it helps to improve their day-to-day condition.

- *Another approach would be to treat the problem as a purely economic one.* Thus, properly functioning markets could solve the problem, and to the extent that there is actually a problem, this indicates that some aspect of the market is not working well. In essence, the logic is that people will buy where they want to live and will take measures, such as insurance, to offset any hazard. The objective might be to make sure that the markets worked through, for example, the provision of information and the availability of appropriate products. This can be challenging as information often fails to inform (see Chapter 7), important values are not catered for in markets, and insurance is not always available (as with flood insurance in much of Australia, or hurricane and wildfire insurance in parts of the US) or is too expensive for those at risk. This approach is similar to one that *places responsibility onto those at risk*.

Recognition of multiple framings and, hence, multiple policy options is not new, and was fundamental to Gilbert White's initial analysis of US flood policy (White, 1945). White argued that the flood problem had to be defined broadly so that the full range of strategies would be considered, rather than the partial approach dominated by major engineering works that resulted from considering flooding purely as a problem of water control.

Each way of framing the problem leads to different objectives and will be at least partially correct in certain circumstances, but may also miss important aspects of the risk. Multiple problem framings may help to ensure that such aspects can be incorporated. In each case, the protection offered is subject to debate: should it be from all threat of the hazard; to some set level (such as the 1:100 or 1 per cent flood);

to some measure related to human safety, such as floodwater depth and velocity; to economic criteria; or simply to levels of awareness among those at risk?

The use of risk management processes may encourage broader approaches; but such processes do not, by themselves, encourage multiple problem framings, although they can accommodate them. This is examined in more detail later in the chapter.

Cause–effect linkages

Most enquiries following major disasters concentrate on institutional issues and preparedness (including the near generic issues of communication, coordination, public education and awareness). Disaster policy research and development research in poorer countries concentrates on social and economic issues, while globally the major research and policy effort is on technological hazards and physical phenomena. Much of the latter is now conducted under the banner of climate change. All three areas often contribute to risk and disasters in ways that are not immediately obvious, and which, through the way the problem is framed are frequently excluded from consideration by emergency and disaster-related policy. They are reviewed briefly below.

Institutional predispositions to disaster

Work on institutional predispositions to disaster examines factors within institutions and organizations (such as major industrial plants, or systems such as transport or energy, that may lead to disasters), and, secondly, aspects of institutions that encourage or discourage disaster resilience by those at risk. The former is often examined in the context of 'safety culture' or 'high reliability organizations' (e.g. Hopkins, 2005). The aviation industry, nuclear power industry and nuclear submarines are examples, at different scales, of high reliability organizations with strong safety cultures. Within the core emergency management sector, the fire services would be seen as having a strong safety culture for their own activities, while a goal of the sector would be to encourage greater adoption of a safety culture throughout society.

Internal to organizations, there are a range of competing theories: Charles Perrow (1984) gained fame through his work on 'normal accidents' and tightly coupled systems. He is pessimistic about our ability to prevent major disasters in complex technological systems. The work of Turner and others on early warnings of failure, on the 'incubation' or gradual pathway to disaster and on safety culture is more optimistic as it specifies elements of institutional culture and behaviour that reduce the likelihood of disaster (Turner, 1978; Turner and Pidgeon, 1997).

Some of the factors found to be important in predisposition to disaster include the absence of effective communication between parts of an organization (silos) and the often related factors of capture by a particular disciplinary, commercial or ideological approach; conflicting intentions or mandates; and an inability, through organizational rigidity or other problems, to take advantage of known precursors or early signals of failure. This may lead to a situation where deviations from design (whether process, activity, structure or object) become accepted as normal instead of being seen as warnings of impending failure.

In summary, attributes predisposing institutions to disaster include:

- relying on stereotypes of what organizational structures and processes should be, rather than acting on the reality of deviations from design and warnings;
- the pressure of work (performance, productivity and time), resulting in safety procedures or failsafe processes being poorly addressed or ignored;
- unclear or confused objectives, such as production deadlines or public relations *versus* precaution or technical feasibility and safety;
- the inability to appreciate or monitor the full extent of the system so that critical parameters are overlooked;
- the issue of learning and blame: it is much easier to blame someone than to make the changes that might be needed for effective learning. Organizations have many opportunities to learn from disasters; however, two common impediments to learning from disasters are information flow, and blame and organizational priorities and politics (Turner, 1978). Organizations often learn the wrong things from an emergency management perspective, such as how to cut corners or reduce costs (e.g. the *Herald of Free Enterprise Report* from the Marine Accident Investigation Branch, undated).

To varying extents, these attributes reflect a failure to think in broad strategic terms beyond immediate pressures and priorities.

When we consider the environment external to specific organizations, our focus is on aspects of institutions that encourage or discourage disaster resilience by those at risk. The institutions of law, local economics and governance, as well as cultural aspects of power, are important in building resilience to disaster. Legal capacity, such as the ability to enforce safety regulations, is also important, as is an institutional environment that fashions patterns of exclusion from sources of power and enterprise, such as the caste system in parts of India, gender divisions in many societies, or the invisibility of undocumented or illegal workers.

It is normal for major societal institutions to give signals that emergency management is a low priority, although this has not been the case with counter-terrorism. This is generally couched in terms of privileging economic development over concerns about natural and technological hazards, and manifests itself as denial or optimism that the potential disaster will not happen for many years.

Social, economic and historical forces

Vulnerable communities exist everywhere – as discussed in Chapter 1 (see Handmer, 2003; Pelling, 2003; Wisner et al, 2004). There is limited agreement on how to measure vulnerability, and it is often asserted that poverty and vulnerability are not the same, largely because poverty is a state, while vulnerability has many components and can change rapidly. Nevertheless, being poor and poorly connected politically, resulting in exclusion from healthcare, sound housing, safety and security, employment opportunities, legal and administrative redress, and other services, is a reasonable first-level surrogate for vulnerability. However, very poor people have taken advantage of sound legal systems, where they are available, and have used the media and political pressure to reduce their vulnerability (Handmer and Monson, 2004; Handmer et al, 2007).

Global trends widely seen as contributing to increased vulnerability by undermining resilience and destroying livelihoods are war and civil strife, and aspects of economic globalization (see O'Keefe et al, 2004; see also the discussion in Chapter 1). Globalized markets and production are creating vast complexes that produce goods and services for wealthier markets. These can be found in many areas of cheap labour, from the call centres of the UK and India, the export factories of Indonesia, Vietnam, and Shenzhen in China, the *maquiladoras* of the US–Mexican border, and the free-trade areas of island states such as Mauritius and Fiji. These complexes provide livelihoods for many people; but in many areas, wages are adequate for survival rather than sufficient to allow the accumulation of wealth, purchase of insurance or other ways of building resilience. In saying this we are aware that this refers to the formal economy. All over the world, and particularly in many African and Asian countries, informal or undocumented economies are expanding strongly, potentially enhancing the real livelihood status of the people involved (Bah and Goodwin, 2003; and see the website International Labour Organization; www.ilo.org).

In wealthier areas, vulnerable communities may emerge as industries close down or shift elsewhere and there is no replacement economic activity. Some areas may be affected by a combination of declining investment and deteriorating infrastructure, with an aging population with associated health and mobility issues, high unemployment and perceptions (if not a reality) of social and political marginalization (e.g. some former coal mining communities in south Wales, UK).

The issue of the extent to which disaster policy should address underlying vulnerabilities and seek to build community resilience, or focus on specific mitigation strategies, is discussed in Chapter 6. For many countries, a general approach dedicated to enhancing resilience through improving access to healthcare, employment security, improved housing and sanitation, etc. has a definite and immediate payoff with costs that can be shared, while the benefits from specific counter-disaster measures are contingent on an event, and on appropriate maintenance and procedures. Research by the Merseyside (UK) fire service showed that fires were closely related to socio-economic status: the more the service worked on the underlying causes of fires, the more it confronted issues of poverty and exclusion (McGurk, 2005).

The physical environment

It is a central theme of this book that so-called 'natural' disasters result from the interaction of human activities with the natural environment, with the resilience of the human activities the most significant component of this interaction and, importantly, the part we have direct influence over. There are at least three ways in which the natural environment can surprise us:

1   with very large natural events, such as the 2004 Boxing Day tsunami; at the national scale there are many examples (e.g. Hurricane Katrina in New Orleans and the 1999 Sydney hailstorm);

2   through the movement of people or activities into more environmentally

challenging areas (e.g. as people move to the coast and warmer cyclone-prone areas, or vast squatter or informal settlements in many third world cities located in previously vacant areas prone to floods and landslides);

3   through environmental change, shifts or variation in climate or weather extremes, which alter the hazard, such as the long drought and strong warming trend in south-eastern Australia and substantial increase in the wildfire season's length, severity and risk of mega-fires (large, uncontrollable and very destructive wild-fires), or destruction of natural resources on which people depend.

Since we cannot predict these surprises (or at least not precisely enough to plan ahead), policy makers need to be aware that the residual (unmanaged) risk may be very large, and disaster management will depend to a significant extent on the quality of emergency management, precautionary fail-safe measures and the resilience of those at risk.

Pervasive uncertainty

The fact that uncertainty is a dominant theme of emergency management is reinforced by the above review of the many ways of framing policy problems and the complexity of cause–effect linkages. The very existence of the emergency management sector is an explicit recognition that we cannot eliminate uncertainty. Emergency management is one of society's fundamental approaches to dealing with the risks and uncertainties arising from technology, nature, culture and lifestyle.

Emergency managers have to make decisions about what to do in the face of uncertainty. There is nothing unusual about this compared to other fields of endeavour, except that for emergency managers decisions often carry very high stakes and are often in the public domain. This visibility makes it difficult to follow tried-and-tested approaches to dealing with the negative outcomes of uncertainty – to hide mistakes or shift blame. Occasionally (perhaps often), emergency managers have to make decisions with high stakes in the near complete absence of information. This absence can sometimes be at least partly resolved through collecting information in the form of data or local intelligence. Yet, often the uncertainty cannot be resolved and may even extend to the possibility that well-intended actions may worsen the situation. Unlike many other areas of policy and management, emergency managers can rarely wait for more information, but must act.

The fundamental question for emergency management is whether to embrace, deny or seek to reduce uncertainty, generally through collecting information. However, frequently time is limited. What other policy domains have minutes or, perhaps at best, hours to assess situations, make life or death decisions, communicate clearly, and then be subject to intense public evaluation – and likely with no chance for correction? The formal, high-profile inquiries following flooding in the UK and Europe (see Bye and Horner, 1998) and fires in Australia (see Doogan, 2006) illustrate the extent and seriousness of this pressure. The uncertainty attached to events is not the only form faced by emergency managers. They also face uncertainties associated with treatment by the mass media, interagency rivalry, potential legal liability, tensions between headquarter management and field operations, and shifts in government priorities and resource availability.

The burgeoning security industry may be better able to cope with uncertainty and negative outcomes by being able to shelter behind the twin shields of national security and commercial confidentiality, both of which are powerful ways of making uncertainty irrelevant or at least obscured. For some, such concealment of uncertainty might be viewed as a positive, allowing decisions to be made without accountability or threats of liability, poor media coverage and the potential impact on careers. For others, it may be viewed as unaccountable, inviting poor decision-making and working against learning from experience.

Expanding what we mean by uncertainty

Since knowledge is never perfect and is frequently ignored, discredited, distorted or subverted, a number of points follow. Uncertainty (or, more broadly, ignorance; see Smithson, 1989, 1991) is pervasive throughout society, and there are many different types of uncertainty and ways of thinking about the subject. Problems will be framed and decisions made according to the degree and type of uncertainty, but often not in an explicit manner.

Probabilistic approaches dominate work on natural and technological risk and hazards, and in the financial sector. Chaos theory and fuzzy logic are well known non-probabilistic approaches to uncertainty. Approaches to uncertainty in fields such as politics, law or medicine are qualitative in character, such as the 'burden of proof' concept in law and the verbal qualifiers used in medicine, such as 'reasonable medical certainty'. Advocates of fuzzy approaches note that everyday language deals with uncertainty via verbal qualifiers characterized as vague or fuzzy (see Smithson, 1991).

Dovers and Handmer (1995) draw on the work of Smithson (1989; 1991) to suggest a three-way classification for policy-framing purposes:

1   *Apparently reducible ignorance*, which can, given sufficient resources, be reduced to inform decisions within useful time frames. Depending on the nature of the problem, information including that produced by science helps to reduce the uncertainty here.
2   *Irreducible ignorance*, which cannot be usefully reduced within the time frames available, either because we are unaware of its existence, lack the necessary capacity or because its attributes (e.g. natural randomness) make it unknowable. This will usually be treated as residual risk, although risk control mechanisms are also often used here if we are aware of these components of the risk.
3   *Self-generated ignorance* arising from human systems, typically via inconsistent policies or laws, deemed irrelevance or taboos, or deliberately through deceit and distortion (often referred to as deviance). This is also part of residual risk, but is often invisible either deliberately through concealment or simply as a result of being ignored.

All three categories are important in most complex policy problems, particularly regarding confusion between the first and second categories, where optimism is typically displayed over the ability to reduce ignorance or uncertainty, and where admissions of ignorance in political or professional terms are nearly taboo. Category three is also very important to unpack simply because it is frequently the least recognized. Nevertheless, category three also houses many of the assumptions and agendas of the stakeholders in risk and emergency management, and many institutional perversities and barriers.

Attributes of emergency management policy problems

As emphasized earlier, a key attribute of emergencies and disasters is uncertainty, although clearly the amount and type of uncertainty will vary from easily identifiable and manageable to being so large that the problem defies clear definition. Uncertainty is one of a vast array of dimensions and challenges presented by emergencies and disasters. These dimensions can be thought of as attributes. Different attributes are likely to suggest different policy approaches, or different mixes of approaches, as reliance on one approach is most unlikely to cope with the full range of challenges. This suggests that some classification or typology of disasters or emergencies is necessary to help with the development of appropriate policy. To help inform a typology of policy problems, we first set out some attributes of the *policy* problems and some attributes related to management and response. These are distinct from the key issues for strategic emergency management that were identified in Chapter 1:

- *Scale* can be considered in three ways. First, some 'events' may be so extensive or complex in space and time that they resist attempts to place spatial or temporal boundaries around them. Second is magnitude or severity – the Asian tsunami was a mega event by any criteria; but even small radiological or biological contamination threats may challenge every aspect of emergency management. Third is potential impacts/loss: economic, livelihoods, ecological, social and institutional. We are good at counting people and buildings, but poor at economic impacts and worse on social, institutional, cultural and longer-term ecological impacts that are often far more significant than immediate losses. Reversibility is part of this attribute.
- *Uncertainty, complexity and surprise* exist with regard to boundaries of where and when, magnitude, adequacy of preparedness and response strategies, coping ability or resilience (including redundancy), and appropriate policy and management options. Complexity is used in both its common meaning of 'complicated' and its scientific meaning of 'complex systems' – regarding causes, pathways, interdependencies, uncertainties and indeterminacies.
- *Visibility* (including immediacy and topicality) of the threat or event is inherent in different disaster or risk types, but is also frequently defined by media and political interests.

Other attributes are more directly related to management:

Table 5.1 *Emergency management typology by attributes*

Attribute typology	Scale	Uncertainty	Visibility	Problem-solving approach	Management attributes (e.g. tractability)
Routine	Modest and well defined in space and time. Minimal impact	Known and quantified	Recognized, but low visibility	'Applied science'	Known, anticipated and well practised
Non-routine	May be large, but defined	Known, but less quantified	High visibility	'Professional consultancy'	Medium; some planning
Complex	Large and/or ill defined in space and time. High impact. Possibly irreversible	Large or unknown in many dimensions. May not be quantifiable	Often very high profile, with intense and long-lasting political and media interest	'Post-normal science'	Low; often well outside previous experience

Source: the 'Problem solving approach' column is adapted from Funtowicz and Ravetz (1993)

- *Conflicting/unclear objectives* as emergency management (and public safety) objectives are often placed in opposition to development and commercial imperatives and practice, and occasionally to political ideologies. Different agencies involved in emergency management may have conflicting views on how the task is best approached.
- *Institutional* issues in the sense of coordination, capacity, trust and legitimacy are central to success in risk management and risk communication, and in terms of institutional clarity and responsibility. It must be clear who has responsibility not simply for leading response, but for planning and policy development.
- *The ability to cope/tractability* will depend on the type of emergency, and the organizations and sophistication of understanding involved. Emergency management organizations cope well with many emergencies. There are, however, exceptions, even for the best resourced groups. In many jurisdictions, the ability to cope is, to varying degrees, dependent on outside assistance. Tractability will vary with the type of emergency and the institutions taking the lead, and will change with time.

A typology of disasters and emergencies

This list of attributes could be detailed further, and there are many ways of representing them; however, most of the main dimensions are captured. When applied to a variety of emergencies, attributes will take the form of continuums from, for example, minor impacts well within the capacity of existing structures to impacts that clearly overwhelm response capabilities; from well-documented and agreed approaches on management to considerable debate on dealing with the problem; from a reasonably unified approach across society to a maze of apparently conflicting priorities; or from straightforward links between cause and effect to unclear and complex origins in social and economic systems.

Drawing on these attributes, we suggest that emergencies can, as a usable first approximation, be placed in three categories as shown in Table 5.1 and explained below: routine, non-routine and complex. Each category is defined with an explanation of the implications for the approach adopted by emergency management.

In summary, the attributes of *routine* emergencies will generally be at the lower end of the attribute continuums, while *complex* emergencies are characterized by attributes at the higher, more difficult, end of the continuums. *Non-routine* emergencies lie in between. Here, most attention is devoted to the third category of emergencies – complex – as this poses the most challenges. There could be more categories; but the intermediate classes would be difficult to distinguish clearly. The classification unintentionally illustrates the issue of language – the same term is sometimes used to describe an event whether it is 'routine' or 'the largest ever'. For example, the term 'flood' covers every event, from a centimetre-deep surface flow with nuisance value to an inundation of Biblical proportions, which threatens a regional economy (wildfires provide similar examples).

The typology reflects a categorization of policy problems by Dovers (2005) and also draws on an emergency management interpretation of the three-way classification developed by Funtowicz and Ravetz (1993), provided by Tarrant (2006). Funtowicz and Ravetz's (1993) work places problems where values are central, facts are in dispute, stakes and uncertainty are high and there is little agreement about what to do within a category that demands a form of understanding and knowledge that they term 'post-normal science' (PNS). Their other categories are 'professional consultancy', applicable to non-routine problems, and 'applied (or normal) science' applicable to routine problems. PNS problems are typically situations where there is conflict over how to approach a risk or even over how to define the risk. Where the physical dimensions of the risk are well defined and agreed on, the response and event management may take the form of a PNS problem, as with Hurricane Katrina.

Routine

These emergencies are reasonably well-defined events, and the likelihood of their occurrence, although not the precise timing, is understood. There is general agreement on what the problem is and on what should be done. The emergencies are seen as part of normal experience (though not normal in the sense used by Perrow, 1984). Organizations are created and trained to deal with these events on a regular basis (e.g. moderate storm damage, predictable river flooding, small bush and structure fires, small and medium contamination incidents, and road accidents). In most developed and many developing countries, these emergencies are coped with well.

The approach

Response will be well rehearsed, well practised or habitual, and guided by standard procedures and rules. The demands on knowledge would correspond with 'applied science' in the Funtowicz and Ravetz (1993) classification. The approach used for such events can usually be characterized as anticipatory: the events are expected although timing may be uncertain – routine events are the bread and butter of emergency management. As a result, they can be, and usually are, fully planned for and quite tractable. The policy emphasis and objectives for this type of problem are typically on eliminating the causes of the problem as far as practicable, or on sharing and shifting the risk (e.g. to commercial insurers) so that social and economic impacts are reduced.

The strategic challenge is to enhance interagency cooperative capacity, and to work on prevention and ways of sharing and shifting the risk. In one sense, policy should work to expand what is treated as routine. Important strategies are engagement with those at risk and appropriate institutional and policy design.

Non-routine

These events are generally anticipated and may have generic plans; but they stretch the emergency system, and require some shifts in operational procedures and thinking through more-than-expected scale, complexity and/or uncertainty. They include multi-vehicle accidents, major storm and cyclone damage, larger fires, substantial contamination incidents and mass casualty events.

The approach

Flexibility and adaptability are called for in response and prevention. Prevention is useful even though the problems are large and often complex since they are generally within the range of experience. Judgement is required between competing priorities, often with multiple agencies and jurisdictions involved.

The knowledge needs required for non-routine problems correspond with the 'professional consultancy' category in the PSN framework, drawing on well-established practice, but including judgement and multiple information inputs. Again, most well-resourced jurisdictions cope with these emergencies, although they will usually exceed the day-to-day coping capacity of emergency service organizations and require help from groups not normally involved with emergencies, as well as assistance from other countries. Poorly resourced and trained jurisdictions may find that for them, non-routine emergencies take on some of the attributes of 'complex emergencies', such as the complexity and uncertainty of appropriate planning and response, potentially resulting in emergency management organizations being over-whelmed and forced into a reactive mode.

The strategic challenges are for policy to shift non-routine problems towards the routine, and to do this in a cost-effective way. A major impediment is that this might require a level of redundancy that is not tolerated in an environment dedicated to eliminating margins as waste and inefficiency. One approach is to re-conceptualize this in terms of well-argued 'failsafe' mechanisms and procedures, rather than the harder-to-argue maintenance of surplus capacity.

Complex emergencies

With complex emergencies, a fundamental issue is that in a context of very large and unknown uncertainty, risk definition and the identification of appropriate strategies are difficult, in part because actions may worsen rather than reduce the risk or, at the very least, may miss the mark completely. Typically, there will be limited agreement on the definition and cause of the problem, as well as on the problem boundaries: indeed, the problem and consequences may be unbounded. Agreement on appropriate action will therefore also be difficult. It is likely that the problem is not amenable to rapid solution, and it is more a case of developing longer-term strategies for risk reduction through containment and consequent management. Table 5.2 lists some of the attributes of complex emergencies.

More conceptually, a risk or problem is said to be *complex* when it exists in several system dimensions at once (e.g. natural, social, political and cultural systems). When problems are complex, destructive multi-system consequences become evident throughout systems and sectors (e.g. an outbreak of foot-and-mouth disease in a previously unaffected country, affecting trade, tourism and farming sectors). A risk is *unbounded* when it is impossible to fence it off from non-problem domains on the grounds that they are irrelevant to the problem (note that this does not mean that the problems are necessarily infinite in time or space, although they may be in terms of our decision-making processes). Even when problems are not obviously global, they can hit us anywhere – the emotional impact of terrorism, the pursuit of compensation in jurisdictions outside of the event (e.g. Bhopal), expansion of regulations or best practice globally (e.g. transport, nuclear energy, dam safety and industrial accidents), or in governmental and non-governmental aid. There is likely to be disruption in many domains, as opposed to risks that are well bounded and controlled, such as car crash fatalities. They are the emergency management equivalent of 'post-normal science' problems, arising when the consequences are substantial, when knowledge is limited and when values, rather than quantifiable expectations, are more relevant, thus demanding quite different forms of knowledge capacities.

The approach

Standard approaches to risk management have difficulty with unbounded risks. One approach is to use probabilities to describe the uncertainty. But we believe that this widely applied approach may be misleading in circumstances where the risk resists clear definition. In some cases, risk treatments may have serious counterintuitive and unintended consequences when the nature of the problem cannot be captured quantitatively but efforts concentrate only on aspects that can be represented in that way.

Since we are dealing here with events and problems that have not always been identified, and have uncertain but very extensive impacts, anticipatory approaches are not possible except in the sense of generic planning. Attempts at precise preparation will likely be overwhelmed by events. The emphasis is on building more resilient communities, institutions and systems underlying response. Clear and strong leadership is required, capable of facilitating and coordinating resources from all sectors of society. Command and control may not be an appropriate approach given the very large uncertainties and practical and conceptual difficulties in 'controlling' ill-defined problems. The strategic challenge is quite different and much greater than for more routine problems.

Complex emergencies may be very large and complex simply because of their size and the number of organizations, jurisdictions and people involved, and the media and political attention that they attract. Their characteristics may merge with those of *complex unbounded problems* (CUPs): when can a risk or problem be said to be complex and unbounded? A recent study identified criteria that describe the attributes of CUPs. These are set out in an indicative way in Table 5.2 to help frame policy and institutional response so that it suits the problem. Taken together, they argue for a high degree of flexibility and adaptability, negotiation between multiple stakeholders at multiple scales, and an awareness of different types of uncertainty and their implications.

Compensation is another key issue: can the event be compensated for and is it insurable? The global insurance industry talks of 'mega-perils' that may be unbounded. Insurers are increasingly concerned about natural hazards and global environmental change, with the US insurance industry, for example, gradually restricting cover for wildfires and hurricanes.

Table 5.2 *Attributes of complex unbounded problems emerging at the more difficult end of 'complex' emergency management problems*

Uncertainties (boundaries)
- Uncertainties are high or unknown, and the event may be unexpected (a surprise).
- Boundaries cannot be localized in space or time.
- The event may be driven by the interaction of processes on multiple time scales.
- The magnitude and consequences of the event may be extreme, but not predictable.
- Important features of the event may resist quantification.

Knowledge, impacts and management
- Knowledge, capacity and responses cannot easily be generalized from one problem to another.
- The full impacts and course of the event depend on choices taken/not taken while the event unfolds.
- Even if the event is foreseen, it is unclear what measures can be taken to prevent or prepare for it.
- The causes of impacts may be counterintuitive.
- Mitigation efforts may make the problem worse.
- The outcome of the event may effectively be irreversible.
- The event may be unprecedented and novel to those experiencing and dealing with it.

Values and experts
- Due to uncertainty, complexity and lack of quantification, there may be no clear delineation between 'experts' and 'non-experts'.
- In the absence of mutual understanding, value issues may be central to viewing the problem or to selecting responses.

Source: Handmer and Proudley (2005)

Complex unbounded problems are the nightmares of emergency management and of communities and governments. Their unpredictability and scale challenge the best of intentions and the most well thought-through preparations. Likely to increase in future for reasons discussed in previous chapters and revisited in Chapter 9, they suggest increased resilience/reduced vulnerability as prime strategies, consideration of redundancy in capacities and failsafe mechanisms, and a strong focus on the institutional system that will support coping with the unexpected and previously not experienced.

The risk standard

Risk-based approaches are increasingly applied in all areas of society as part of regulatory, commercial and management processes, including emergency management. Are such approaches adequate across the range of types of policy problems? Disagreements about even the most well-documented risks such as smoking and climate change are normal, with many risks offering much more scope for debate, such as flood recurrence intervals or management of landscape-scale wildfire risk. A leading international model, the Australian–New Zealand Risk Management Standard, sees risk in terms of the chance of something happening that will have an impact on objectives (Standards Australia, 2004; see Chapter 3). Many scientists and engineers define risk strictly in terms of the event size by frequency of occurrence using numerical probabilities, and the assumption that risk can be measured objectively underlies much contemporary risk management. But those at risk – the public – emphasize elements of fairness and trust rather than numerical probabilities, while cultural researchers argue that 'it seems more appropriate to view risk as the embodiment of deeply held cultural values and beliefs' (Jasanoff et al, 1995).

Even where there is agreement on the approach taken to risk analysis, it is likely that those involved will have different priorities – for example, commercial establishments in a small tourist town amidst forested mountains may see wildfire as a threat to business income, rather than as a threat to life and property or to wildlife.

This suggests that as the risk management process moves from the routine to grapple with more complex problems, it is properly seen as the subject of negotiation between stakeholders, rather than simply as a definitive, quantified practice. The Australian–New Zealand Risk Management Standard and other risk management protocols (often subdivided into risk assessment, analysis and management) set out a structured process for stakeholders to negotiate what the objectives of emergency management are, the criteria for assessing the risk and what should be done about it (see Figure 5.1 and Figure 3. 1(b) in Chapter 3). To its advocates, it is a powerful tool that greatly broadens the scope of the more traditional approaches of emergency management based on hazard analysis, prevention, preparedness, response and recovery (the terms vary, but the basic steps are the same). The process in most risk analysis and management frameworks is designed to be expansive and inclusive, and can accommodate multiple problem framings through negotiation. The Australian–New Zealand framework has similarities to the frameworks frequently used in policy analysis and development, and is compatible with the policy framework developed for this book, as shown in Chapter 3. It can be used with either quantitative or qualitative information on the risk, although the tendency is to use quantitative data (often implying a greater degree of certainty and knowledge than actually exists, especially where non-routine and complex problems are concerned).

In practice, however, the risk management process is often applied in a mechanistic fashion, thereby potentially subverting some of its advantages. Unfortunately, some variants of this process do not make objective-setting – also known as 'desired outcomes' – fully explicit. This is closely connected with problem definition and framing. In the absence of clear objectives, it may be difficult to develop risk management options that actually deal with the problem; as a result, and importantly, it may not be possible to assess progress. Philosophically, it is unlikely that we can 'manage' everything. Nevertheless, the approach appears to work well with routine and even many non-routine problems, as described earlier. Complex unbounded problems pose much more of a challenge for risk management approaches as generally practised, in part, because of the different types of uncertainties that such problems introduce.

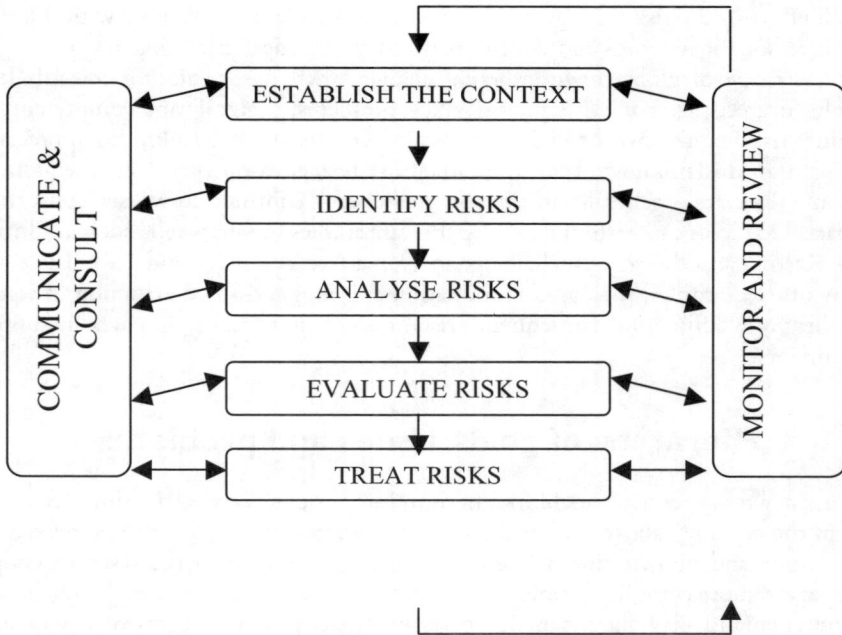

Figure 5.1 *The Australian–New Zealand risk management process*

Note: Most effective use of this process requires explicit objective-setting, recognition of residual risk and incorporation of multiple problem framing.
Source: Standards Australia (2004)

Residual risk

The need to acknowledge and attend to the residual risk is too often downplayed in risk management. This highlights a major weakness from an emergency management perspective, even though the weakness may be viewed as positive from the perspective of land development and other interests. In addition, aspects of the risk can be traded away against emergency management, allowing the risk to be taken. Development may occur in areas subject to floods or other periodic and predictable hazards because emergency management procedures are relied on to facilitate appropriate safety and damage-reducing behaviour. Buildings can be constructed to certain standards and warning systems can be installed to take care of the residual risk. This is not to deny the utility of such negotiated approaches; but it should be recognized that the result will often be residential and critical utility development in what (to emergency management) are high-risk areas, and that symptoms rather than causes of vulnerability are being addressed.

There are other categories of residual risk that are less obvious and are frequently overlooked in policy. Some of these exist now and more will emerge in the future.

Much effort in the risk management arena, understandably, deals only with the risk that is reasonably obvious and which exists today, although increasing acknowledgement is made of global environmental change, with its orientation towards less visible future risks. For most major policy problems, a significant component of residual risk is unknown or highly uncertain (Dovers, 1995). Failure to appreciate and plan for this 'unknown zone' of residual risk is one reason why the consequences of some disasters – generally in the complex class – continue to worsen long after impact. Examples can be found among the case studies in Chapter 1, such as Hurricane Katrina and the refugee challenge in Goma (see Boxes 1.1 and 1.8). There are many other examples, such as contamination episodes and the destruction of water supplies by wildfire, and consequent erosion and water quality impacts in supply catchments.

Hierarchy of goals, issues and problems

Emergency management capabilities need to be considered across the three levels set out in the typology above. The tendency is for performance criteria to be related to the routine and non-routine, while ignoring the capabilities of the system to cope with larger, more complex, problems and events. These events pose a major challenge as they demand very significant increases in capacity in all aspects of emergency management and that capacity is often not forthcoming in an environment determined to eliminate any excess capacity, unless it can be reframed as a security issue.

To bring some of this material together, we draw from the example of community resilience. Table 5.3 summarizes and offers comparison with the social goals of sound emergency management and adaptation to climate change. In this hierarchy, the social goal is resilience, and the point is to illustrate that even a complex unbounded problem can be broken into a set of (albeit complicated) tractable tasks:

- *Social goal:* resilience.
- *Complex unbounded problem*: building resilience in excluded, marginalized groups to the extent that they have maximum reasonable capacity to cope with disturbance.
- *Non-routine problem*: livelihood security following disaster.
- *Routine problems*:
  - aid that stimulates the local economy;
  - emergency management that protects local livelihoods;
  - managing long-term recovery;
  - emergency management staff focused on assets and evacuation;
  - livelihoods not part of emergency management objectives;
  - economic efficiency and commercial objectives that undermine the local economy.

Such an analysis could be repeated taking many pathways, all addressing the same higher-levels goals and problems. In Chapter 6, we examine policy development and implementation, including the question of policy instrument choice.

Table 5.3 Hierarchy of goals, issues, problems and instruments

	Goal		
	Resilience	**Sound emergency management**	**Climate change adaptation**
Issue	Poor resilience; limited recovery after disaster in disadvantaged communities and sectors	Uneven performance of emergency management	Escalating number and severity of natural events
Problem	Ensuring livelihood security after disasters – a non-routine problem (ensuring aid flows)	Reduce impact and consequences of disaster – likely to be routine (manage the physical phenomena and obvious impacts)	A complex unbounded problem
Principle	Local economic vitality (equity in access to services and economic opportunity; legal rights approach)	Equity in distribution of risk (uniform standard of emergency management; targeting areas most in need or where the impact of improved emergency management would be greatest)	Maintaining economic productivity and the pattern of distribution (ensuring that adaptation is part of existing programmes for emergency management and planning)
Instruments (see Chapter 6)	Generic (e.g. local economic development)	Hazard specific (e.g. warning systems, flood walls)	Generic and specific measures

Note: Alternative framings are set out early in this chapter; the different framings are not necessarily incompatible.

Conclusion

This chapter has stressed the importance of closely considering the way in which problems are defined: the policy actors involved, the information needed and the responses suggested will all be affected by this. We have also emphasized the fact that defining the problem will depend on the perspective of those involved; hence, multiple problem framings should be recognized and utilized to inform problems – it is doubtful that any framing is unjustified in terms of perceived risk. The discussion now turns to policy formulation and implementation.

6

Responding to the problem:
Policy formulation and implementation

Once policy problems have been defined, the issue becomes one of how best to achieve the aims of the policy. In order to achieve results, mechanisms are required to implement policy. These mechanisms are developed and applied within particular policy styles that may emphasize, for example, voluntary cooperation or legal sanctions. This chapter covers key issues dealing with the choice of policy approach, and the selection and implementation of policy instruments. It does not go into detail on all available instruments, but rather provides an overview of policy instruments and styles, and draws on indicative examples.

The chapter first examines a broader question of balance in emergency management: whether to focus on specific strategies or on generic resilience, and the choices these directions entail. It then discusses issues of adaptability and flexibility, before going on to survey policy instruments and their suitability for the kinds of problems characterized in Chapter 5. Lastly, it considers implementation.

Broad policy choice: Generic resilience or specific instruments?

Emergency management is increasingly a process where trade-offs between the often conflicting objectives of hazard reduction, economic use, social values and the environmental amenity of a hazardous area are negotiated explicitly. The implicit admission is that we are 'managing' rather than 'preventing' exposure to hazards, or reducing risk rather than eliminating it, and accommodating multiple social goals in the process. This requires additional skills: those of the negotiator rather than the builder or commander are increasingly called for. Results of broader thinking include developing commitment to, and local capacity for, a broad range of policy instruments, including modifying the legal liability environment, managing community vulnerability, and involving lending institutions and insurers. This raises the issue of whether we can or should try to 'manage' everything.

Given limited resources, should we implement short-term measures that focus directly on the hazard, such as education and flood walls, or build longer-term community resilience through wealth generation and improved livelihood security? The need for spare capacity – the safety margin provided by redundancy – was highlighted in Chapter 1, as was the difficulty of achieving this in a political age where the trend is towards eliminating margins, rather than providing some surplus capacity. Inevitably, this means that resources have to be taken from one activity and moved to emergency management when needed. This happens, to a certain extent, during response and recovery – and is unavoidable and appropriate in large events – but rarely occurs in planning or prevention.

Concentrating solely on measures to alleviate the impacts of specific disasters is unlikely to address the avoidable causes of disaster, even though many such measures alleviate the symptoms of disaster and have high political credibility – and rightly so given that they save lives and property. They may also sometimes be the only solution, other than emigration, such as with sea walls and gates protecting villages against tsunamis in Japan, and other very hazardous environments. Adaptive capacity exists in most communities; but it is unlikely to have been developed solely for natural hazards except where hazards dominate people's lives. Promoting resilience, and adaptive communities and emergency management agencies, will require attention to many areas of society, including areas normally seen as well outside the ambit of emergency management policy. Thus, a choice in favour of generic resilience frames emergencies and disasters as part of a necessarily whole-of-government and society endeavour, not a policy concern contained within a limited range of specialist agencies. A choice in favour of specific measures targeting known hazards will be simpler and cheaper, and possibly effective as long as events of unexpected magnitude do not occur.

Policies need to consider what undermines resilience or makes people and their livelihoods more vulnerable – in other words, what are the underlying causes or contributors to an increased risk of disaster? If this is not established, we may be attempting to provide a solution to the wrong problem. By its nature, such an approach is strategic and more likely to be part of broader community development than directly related to risk reduction for a specific hazard.

Most hazards are largely invisible and intangible until they are manifested in the extreme events that trigger disasters. Why should they receive priority over the many tangible, visible, immediate and urgent needs of the countries and communities concerned – needs such as security, clean water, housing and employment? This is how the broad policy choice is commonly framed, in a fashion typical of modern policy debates – binary choices and trade-offs in a constrained world. It is better to ask what mix of generic and specific measures is possible, is likely to be effective and is capable of contributing to more than one policy goal – clean water, economic diversity, etc., as well as resilience in the face of potential disasters.

Even when the question of priorities among policy goals is set aside, success is not guaranteed – specific measures must be seen as desirable and supported by those at risk. There is an important difference between having measures in place and success. Implementation of policy can be plagued with individual and organizational deviance, unintended consequences, legal problems, conflict with other social goals and expectations, and changing political or administrative priorities, which may themselves be driven by recent disasters. The same comments can be made about the actual process of measuring success (Handmer, 2000). Implementation is dealt with later in this chapter.

Generic approaches to hazards management

Generic approaches generate the wealth, expertise, communication capacities, infrastructure and other conditions needed for implementing specific strategies, such as building regulations. They may also increase resilience to all hazards through improved building, planning and infrastructure, and by increasing or establishing access to resources in a crisis. Generic measures generally assume effective government, or work to put it in place. But whatever the difficulties, a major advantage of generic approaches is that they serve other, and often multiple, social goals. They are not limited to serving the goal of reducing or managing a specific hazard – important though this might be to those in the field, it is rarely a high priority in poor countries (see, for example, Handmer, 2003a, 2003b). Importantly, the more systematic the policy approach (assuming effectiveness), the less of an issue spare capacity and redundancy becomes, which is more critical where there is reliance on the fewer, more targeted options and resources of a specific hazards approach. Generic human development and capacity-building generally provide communities with a greater range of coping strategies and fall-back resources.

The development literature on hazards and disasters overwhelmingly supports a generic approach, with the emphasis on vulnerability reduction through the development process. For example, the Inter-American Development Bank (CEPAL and BID, 2000) states that 'disasters are clearly a development problem'. Both the United Nations International Decade for Natural Disaster Reduction and its follow-up make the link between disasters and sustainable development, emphasizing the need to reduce vulnerability, to safeguard 'natural and economic resources, and ... social wellbeing and livelihoods' (UN–ISDR, 1999). In its *World Disasters Report 2001*, the International Federation of Red Cross and Red Crescent Societies (IFRC) takes a similar line:

> ... disasters become ever more frequent, aid dollars and development gains are being washed away ... disaster is no longer a brief dip on the curve of development but a danger to the [development] process itself. (IFRC, 2001, p1)

The academic work on this topic goes back into the 1950s; but influential pieces include O'Keefe et al's 1976 paper in *Nature* and the late Fred Cuny's book *Disasters and Development* (1983), with its emphasis on broad development issues. The links between disasters and development (and, during more recent times, sustainable development) are not confined to developing countries. The theme of the summary report of the US second assessment of natural hazards emphasizes generic issues and, in particular, the integration of hazard management with sustainable development (Mileti, 1999). Very importantly, the UN's *Hyogo Framework for Disaster Prevention*

– agreed to by 168 countries at the UN's Second Conference on Disaster Reduction at Kobe in 2004 – emphasizes the point in its first Priority Action, which states: 'promote and integrate disaster risk reduction into development programming' (UN–ISDR, 2004).

Generic measures fall loosely into two categories, both dedicated to resilience:

1 those that strive to build resilience through the development process, and sometimes by resolving serious impediments to social and economic advancement, such as systematic violence;
2 those that are multi-hazard, such as education for safety, or that tackle global environmental change.

Many of the issues addressed by generic measures were set out in Chapter 1. Half of the global population including many in otherwise rich countries, are largely preoccupied with the challenges of their day-to-day existence: food; health, including HIV-AIDS; potable water; and livelihood security, among other issues. Clearly, people and communities in these circumstances are likely to have priorities that concern improving livelihood security, ending war and violence, and creating opportunities for their children. For example, people without an income flow may not be able to either prepare for or recover from a disaster; well-sited, well-built housing protects its occupants in contrast to poorly sited, low-quality dwellings; those who do not have enough to eat normally will find their options limited when the existing food supply is interrupted. They may view expensive specific hazard mitigation as a waste of resources and unrelated to their needs. Addressing the priorities set out above should improve resilience for a wide variety of emergencies. This is not restricted to developing countries; most countries contain substantial groups whose social and economic status forces day-to-day survival priorities.

Specific approaches to hazards management

Specific approaches are those dedicated solely to mitigating a particular hazard and which have no other intentional purpose. They have saved many lives and countless amounts of property damage. Shelters designed to provide safe havens from sea flooding, for example, have saved thousands in Orissa, India (Sparrow, 2001); cyclone warning systems in the Pacific provide timely warnings to poor small island countries; thousands of flood-resistant houses provide protection in Vietnam (Jaquemet, 2001); and earthquake, wind and fire building codes in many countries similarly protect households and businesses. Major levee or dike systems protect the populations of many countries against sea and river flooding. The Netherlands may present the extreme case, where dikes keep the sea out and allow the nation to flourish. However, levees may also increase vulnerability, and when they gave way in The Netherlands and the US (in New Orleans and elsewhere), the consequences were thousands of deaths and massive property damage.

Opportunities for promoting and implementing specific approaches present themselves in various ways (see the discussion of 'Policy and institutional learning:

Purposes and forms' in Chapter 7):

- immediately following a disaster when these measures have high priority, as well as public support;
- where there are organizations whose mission includes the use of specific tools, such as engineering works and public education;
- when local people demand action in the face of perceived risks;
- when the institutional context would enable and support low-cost measures, such as minor changes to building techniques that can often result in large improvements and locally based warning systems, which are an underused, low-cost measure.

Important constraints and qualifications surrounding specific approaches and measures include the following:

- Measures are often given low priority by governments and the public so that those at risk must be involved and support the measure.
- Measures divert scarce resources from other priorities, which may be perceived as more socially and politically urgent.
- Measures may not address underlying causes of vulnerability, but only mitigate the impacts of events.
- Occasionally, measures and approaches may make the situation worse – for example, by increasing vulnerability to other hazards or by providing a false sense of security so that important complementary measures are overlooked.

Emergency management agencies tend to favour specific approaches – that is their mandate. They may also be limited by the problem framing and institutional division of roles that do not see disasters as a human development issue. However, in poorer countries, those at risk see the generic or macro-issue of livelihood security as key to their resilience.

The differences between the two general approaches may not be as significant as it first appears. Often, the two approaches are intertwined, with many specific approaches depending on the right generic or institutional conditions for their success.

For crisis response: Flexibility and adaptability

Strategic policy work is about trying to shape the future. Yet, by definition, the future is unknowable. Reconciling this apparent paradox is the task less of the emergency manager than of the disasters and emergency policy and institutional system within which the manager operates.

Developing and rehearsing a range of scenarios is a fundamental tool for framing the future and for establishing the relationships and generic plans needed for major events. Generic plans include mass (and specific types of casualties, such as burns) casualties; communications; media; evacuation or sheltering options;

transport; energy; search and rescue; radiological and other contaminants; visits by dignitaries; how to manage political pressure; and so on. However, even very well-resourced scenarios and plans can fail in spectacular fashion, as with Hurricane Katrina in New Orleans. The political and media circumstances may be such that failure is almost unnoticed. Alternatively, emergency managers may feel blamed for natural phenomena and pushed into action that, while politically useful, does little to help the people (as with much international post-impact disaster aid or some mass evacuations). This is another reminder that emergency managers, unlike their colleagues in most other areas of public policy, are faced with having to make urgent, critical binary decisions to do one thing or another with no other option, scope for delay or compromise, and which may be difficult to reverse.

Plans, scenarios and exercises are a guide. They are not reality, although occasionally (especially with smaller more routine events) the event and response will unfold as expected and planned for. One of the major challenges for emergency managers is to accept the limitations of the planning and preparedness tools. As just mentioned, apart from smaller events, these tools should be seen as a means to an end – that is, to develop the relationships and mindsets needed for the management of major events with all the unexpected issues and problems that they bring. They are not ends in themselves. Put another way, planning is a way of making an idea work. Planning 'must be societal [i.e. not an individual activity], future oriented, non-routinized, deliberate [not trial and error], strategic, and linked to action' (Alexander, 1986, p43).

One aim of the planning process is to build a constituency of support for the plan or guidelines. The document (called the plan or guide) should be seen as a record of agreements reached during the process of planning; but with circumstances constantly changing, the document is unlikely to ever be completely up to date. Emergency planning in this way can be viewed as more process than product.

The relationships and decision-making skills developed during planning and complex exercises should form the basis of a flexible, adaptable approach to emergency management. But they will not do this automatically. A critical approach is needed rather than a self-congratulatory one. This may be harder to achieve in an environment increasingly defined by security or counter-terrorism, rather than by public safety from natural and technological threats. One result is that planning and exercises may be closed to external scrutiny. Nevertheless, if trust exists or can be developed across institutions, it may be possible to include a range of perspectives and critical evaluation, while keeping the processes confidential. Failure to include diverse perspectives almost guarantees that the exercises will be predictable and does little to develop the necessary flexibility and adaptive capacity needed to handle future disasters.

By changing and limiting the impact of disaster, emergency management can influence the future. At best, this results in improved resilience and capacities – at worst, in a narrowing of learning possibilities and increased reliance on centralized interventions.

Policy problems and policy instruments

Here, the general types of instruments are set out against the problem classification developed in Chapter 5, guided by the assumption that the nature of the problem should inform the kinds of policy approach and policy instruments chosen.

Minor or routine emergencies

These problems are anticipated and can be planned for in a context of little uncertainty about what is needed. The basic planning and response of all the emergency services is based on a certain amount of spare capacity to cope with the anticipated and regularly occurring events – storms, floods, fires, transport and other accidents, minor toxic spills, etc. Otherwise, there would be almost no ability to respond apart perhaps to minor single events.

Measures typically used for routine emergencies are short- to medium-term measures, including risk analysis and risk treatments generally dedicated to minimizing the occurrence of such events; warning and alarm systems; measures for responding in a standardized way to routine residual risk; and the delivery of assistance by government and NGOs to communities affected by relatively frequent events, such as monsoon flooding in Vietnam or wildfires in Australia and California.

Most communities in better-off parts of the world are able to cope with these emergencies, within limited need for external assistance and intervention. They have enough capacity with their local emergency services, loss redistribution through insurance, and support through established welfare, health and other programmes. Higher-level government involvement is generally needed, however, for comprehensive risk analysis and management, especially where this involves regulations or major incentives to reduce the risk, and in many cases where land-use planning is required. In poorer areas, local people generally cope informally and with outside assistance from their networks, or external NGOs and government, if the event attracts sufficient media attention or the country has existing aid agreements in place for such events.

Risk reduction in the context of routine incidents is relatively straightforward as the dimensions of the risks are usually well understood and solutions are a matter of resources and clear trade-offs.

Non-routine or meso-emergencies

Non-routine emergencies are often anticipated in a general sense, and much of what is written above for 'routine' problems will apply with the following modifications. Non-routine events are often larger and rarer than routine events, and planning is therefore more generic than for routine emergencies. It may involve the application of risk management processes (see Chapter 5), with an emphasis on risk identification and using treatments to reduce the scale of the problem, and on planning for the coordination of resources from multiple sources. Flexibility and adaptability are called for in response and prevention, the capacity of emergency services is stretched during such events, and resources from outside the affected area are likely to be needed. But the problems do not pose overwhelming challenges to existing emergency management policy and practice, or to technological capacities. This category could also include policy processes or decisions across a suite of routine problems, such as establishing a multi-hazard policy process or national floodplain management standards.

Complex unbounded emergencies

The primary attributes of these low probability but very high consequence emergencies are uncertainty combined with complexity across most dimensions. Appropriate policy instruments should be longer-term ones dedicated to societal and economic resilience, with incorporation of the precautionary principle and, thus, more proactive approaches, where appropriate, in contrast to the anticipatory measures suitable for more routine risks. Options include long-term planning instruments to avoid hazardous areas and to reduce the vulnerability of infrastructure and buildings, and institutional measures such as insurance and improved livelihood security. In terms of explicit planning, it would generally be government that would need to take the lead. There is often limited interest from other sectors due to the uncertainties involved, which may make the risk seem irrelevant or someone else's problem. The long time periods between occurrences of such events are very often outside the planning and accountability horizons of many organizations. Occasionally, the opposite occurs, with people at risk very concerned about the problem, such as with radioactive or other contamination. If commercial processes or products are involved, companies will often work to undermine any attempt at control or management (see, for example, the European Environment Agency's report *Late Lessons from Early Warnings*, 2001).

Response will need maximum flexibility and adaptability, and would have to provide the needed leadership to make decisions, harness society's resources and have the capacity to expand critical facilities, such as casualty care, identification and handling of the dead, and transportation and rationing of food supplies. This is especially critical: even if there is spare capacity, it is unlikely to be sufficient to make a difference. The gap in capacity will have to be filled by harnessing all of society's resources – government, commercial, civil society and international assistance. Recovery planning for coordination of resources, rather than command and control, is the key as normal response capacity will almost always be overwhelmed. Institutional capacity for adaptability and for whole-of-government and whole-of-society response is needed (see Chapter 8).

Policy instruments and styles of implementation

Having well-developed policy statements will not make any difference by themselves, apart from changes in commitment, anticipation or expectation – a policy avows intent. The policy must be implemented, which may include monitoring for compliance and means of enforcing compliance. Typically, an agency or higher-level government authority develops policy that requires officials, lower levels of government or the public to actually implement it. The challenge is how to achieve implementation (see May et al, 1996). In the hazards and disaster domain, policy implementation style can be classified into three classes known simply as:

1 *coercion* (e.g. through regulations and threats of punitive measures) and instruments, which in the general policy literature are termed regulatory instruments;
2 *cooperation* (e.g. financial incentives, assistance with planning or negotiating trade-offs to accommodate multiple objectives), termed more generally as incentive or collaborative instruments; and
3 *exhortation, guidance or sermonizing* (such as public education and information provision), otherwise known as moral suasion or educative instruments.

A more comprehensive range of policy classes and instruments is given in Table 6.1, which indicates both the difference and the blurred boundaries between the three categories above. Table 6.1 indicates the richness of options available and is a useful aide memoir for policy analysis and design. It also indicates a fundamental point: arguments over particular instruments and their general qualities are usually futile. Policy-makers and policy communities have at their disposal many instruments, all of which will be useful in different situations and combinations. And we can remind ourselves that *all instruments are forms of information, aimed at changing individual or collective behaviours*. Whether the 'message' is a threat, a plea, an incentive or disincentive, or a signpost, policy instruments are messages. A massive tax impost, crippling fine or a prison sentence are all threatening messages, whether considered market or legal mechanisms. An educational instrument may be subtle and respectful; or it may rely on shocking and confrontational images, as some health programmes do. Choosing policy instruments is a matter of choosing the most appropriate medium for the message in a given situation. Viewed in this way, policy instrument choice invites a more objective comparative analysis, rather than an argument over, for example, the relative merits in a broader sense of economic versus legal instruments.

The rest of this chapter focuses largely on the level of broad categories (detailed discussion of each specific instrument requires considerably more space than provided in this volume and is context dependent). The consideration of a detailed menu of instruments and the basis for selecting from this menu (see Table 6.1) is, nevertheless, encouraged.

Although detailed, the menu in Table 6.1 is, nonetheless, still a summary. As the middle column indicates, each of the broad classes contains multiple options, only some of which are identified here. These within-class options are often very different and invite close consideration. For example, among market mechanisms, the disincentive of a tax impost is different from the positive incentive of a rebate. In training and education, the options, again, vary and are suited to different purposes and groups of people. Education or communication-based programmes are likely to require organizational development, and so on.

While this discussion has been about selecting an instrument, it is usually the case that an *interdependent set of instruments* will be used within a policy programme to achieve stated policy goals. Even when one instrument is the major focus, others

Table 6.1 *A menu of policy instruments for emergencies and disasters*

Class	Selected major instruments	Style
1 Research and monitoring	Increase knowledge in a general or specific sense regarding hazards, vulnerability, success of policy initiatives, community awareness, etc.	Exhortation, cooperation
2 Improving communication and information flow	Aid information flow between research and policy; of policy imperatives to research; between agencies, firms and individuals, and through a wide range of mechanisms, such as indicator systems, community-based monitoring, etc.	Exhortation, cooperation
3 Training and education	General public education and education targeting sub-sets of the community; formal curricula in schools and universities; specific skills development and training.	Cooperation, exhortation
4 Consultation	External mediation over conflicts; negotiation; facilitated planning procedures; dispute resolution; inclusive policy processes.	Cooperation, exhortation
5 Inter-governmental agreements	Intergovernmental agreements/policies, memoranda of understanding, etc. between countries or within countries for cooperation, joint response, information-sharing, etc.	Cooperative, coercion
6 Legal requirements	*Statute law:* statutes or regulations under existing law to create institutional arrangements; establish statutory objects and agency responsibilities; guarantee public rights in policy processes; prohibit certain activities; zone land and control development; define and enforce standards; create penalties. *Common law:* applications of doctrines such as negligence or nuisance to prevent or punish risk-creating behaviours.	Coercion, cooperation
7 Planning and assessment procedures	Incorporation of emergency and disasters in land-use planning and social and environmental impact assessment; mandated risk assessment.	Cooperation, coercion
8 Self-regulation	Incorporation of disaster/emergency considerations within industry or firm codes of practice or ethic, professional standards and recommended procedures.	Cooperation, exhortation

9 Community participation	Community-based risk assessment and management; public participation in higher-level policy formulation; freedom of information laws; rights to comment on development proposals; community monitoring of hazards; joint government– community implementation of programmes.	Cooperation
10 Market and economic aspects	Taxes/charges; use charges; subsidies; rebates; penalties; performance; competitive tendering.	Cooperation, coercion, exhortation
11 Institutional change	New or revised institutional system or organizational features to enable implementation of other instruments.	Cooperation, coercion, exhortation
12 Adjustment of other policies	The assessment and, if necessary, alteration of incentives, goals or processes in other policy settings that increase vulnerability or decrease resilience, or which block desired policy change.	n/a
13 Doing nothing	Inaction is usually seen as a policy failure, but may be justified after reasoned analysis.	n/a

Note: n/a = not applicable.

will be needed to support it. An economic measure will require a legal mandate and a communication strategy. Doing nothing should involve a monitoring programme to assess future needs for action.

The reality of mixed instrument packages leads to an important observation, somewhat at odds with the above claim regarding the equality of instruments as different means of communicating the message. This is that some classes can be considered *universal policy instruments*, always required even if only in a supporting role (see Chapter 8 for additional discussion and Chapter 7 on communication):

- *Legal.* In societies subject to the rule of law, defensibility in law must be considered and catered for, whether through new or existing statute, common or customary law. Management regimes will require statutory competence; market mechanisms will require a legal basis for implementation; and so on. In public policy, instruments must have a legal basis if they are designed to affect existing patterns of behaviour and are expected to survive long.
- *Economic.* In every society, much human and organizational behaviour results from economic incentives or disincentives. In many countries, the primary objective of government is economic growth, which sometimes clashes with the

priorities of emergency management. The importance of economic incentives may be active and positive in policy design (creating incentives or removing disincentives for desired behaviours), or it may be passive and negative (not correcting disincentives for desired behaviours or incentives for undesirable behaviours).

- *Institutional.* In a world where humans only achieve common goals or reconcile difference through institutions, policy interventions can only be agreed to and implemented in a suitable institutional and organizational environment. As with the law, this may already exist or be easily adapted, or it may require major institutional reform (see Chapter 8).
- *Communication.* In any policy field, but especially a whole-of-society one such as disasters, a range of people need to know about the instrument, its purpose and implementation. Thus, communication is a necessary component of any policy package, often with multidirectional information pathways to be created and used.

Policy instrument choice

With such a rich menu of policy instruments available, how does one choose the instrument or mix of instruments in a given situation? This invites the use of a set of criteria for policy instrument choice. However, before dealing with more detailed criteria, the first cut – consistent with the policy approach of 'mixed scanning' (see Chapter 2) – is generally an intuitive or subjective matter. Any individual or, preferably, group of people from the policy community will quickly delete some options on the basis of experience. However, it is desirable that some reference to a complete list of policy options is made in order to guard against the tendency towards the convenient or familiar instrument being immediately and, perhaps, inappropriately favoured.

At a more detailed level, Table 6.2 presents a summary set of criteria to form the basis of a more rigorous comparison of the benefits and costs of alternative policy options, stated as questions to be asked of each alternative. Some criteria can be used in a strongly analytical or quantified manner, whereas others will be applied more qualitatively or subjectively. And, importantly, individual criterion will be more or less critical in different situations, while the art and craft of instrument choice involves a balance and compromise between criteria – no instrument will ever be 'perfect'. These criteria can be used as a basis for discussion, in a more structured comparative matrix, or in a mix of the two.

These criteria have two uses. The first is to aid analysis and discussion of the most suitable policy choice for the purpose at hand. They do not make an answer necessarily obvious or easy; in fact, consideration of multiple criteria will complicate the process. But they do encourage a more sophisticated, defensible and more easily communicated process of choice. The second use arises from the observation that 'perfect' choices are rare and may be the less obvious but more important use of the criteria in Table 6.2. A chosen instrument will rarely score highest on every criterion, but nonetheless may be favoured. A criterion against which an instrument is ranked less well identifies an implementation issue that will require attention. For example,

Table 6.2 *Criteria for selecting policy instrument*

Criteria	Question, relative to other instruments
Dependability	How certain is it that the instrument will lead to the achievement of policy goals?
Timeliness	Can the instrument be designed and applied within the necessary time frame?
Cost and efficiency	What is the likely gross cost and efficiency of the instrument, relative to the stated goals?
Systemic potential	Does the instrument address underlying causes, rather than only direct causes and symptoms of vulnerability?
Information and monitoring requirements	Is the necessary information available to design, implement and monitor the performance of the instrument, or can it be made available?
Distributional impacts	Will implementation of the instrument have uneven or inequitable impacts across the affected population; if so, can these be managed in an acceptable manner?
Political and institutional feasibility	Is proposal and implementation of the instrument feasible in terms of political support and institutional capacity?
Ability to be enforced or avoided	Can implementation/uptake of the instrument be enforced; can it be avoided easily?
Communicability	Can the logic, detail and implementation requirements of the instrument be communicated to those responsible for implementation or affected by it?
Flexibility	Is the instrument capable of being adapted and adjusted in the face of changing circumstances?

if dependability and timeliness are critical criteria in a given situation – quite likely in the disasters field – but communicability and equity implications are criteria that the instrument does not rate highly against, then careful communication and some form of adjustment or compensation package are suggested. Or, if timeliness is not an issue and institutional feasibility a problem, then institutional development may be possible to allow good implementation of a favoured instrument.

A note of realism is required. Policy instrument choice is never a fully rational, objective and measured activity, and social norms and broad policy and political styles will dictate, or at least limit, choices. Even if the careful analysis and recommendation of the policy adviser is overridden by political expediency or in the heat of the disaster moment, at the very least the weaknesses and implementation difficulties of the chosen instrument will be more apparent than they otherwise would. Importantly, the limits of the choice will be a matter of record that may lay the basis for later, more informed, redesign of the policy programme.

Policy styles and attributes required for implementation

Returning to our three general categories of exhortation, cooperation and coercion: coercion and cooperation are known variously as 'carrot or stick', 'incentives or sanctions' or 'persuasion or punishment', while exhortation is also referred to as sermonizing, moralizing, lecturing or moral suasion. Whichever approach is taken – and most often the approach, in practice, is some mixture of all three – those implementing the policy on the ground require certain attributes. These can be seen most simply as follows:

* Those involved must want to do it (i.e. they must have *commitment* to the policy objectives, and that commitment must be matched with a recognized and respected mandate).
* They must have the ability or *capacity* to implement the objectives in terms of human, financial and information resources, as well as organizational capacity.
* Cutting across both these attributes, there should be a *process* to deal with conflicts between the different interest groups – in particular, the actual and perceived conflicts between the imperatives of emergency management, economic development and environmental amenity.

These attributes apply to implementation in many areas outside of emergency management, but are often closely linked (e.g. private-sector regulation, intergovernmental relations and the criminal justice system).

We now consider in a little more detail the three different policy classes (Table 6.3).

Exhortation

This approach is used widely in emergency management, both in circumstances where there is strong political and media support, and where the risk is not highly visible. It is covered in more detail in Chapters 4 and 7. Most preparedness and planning rely on exhortation through awareness-raising and education programmes. The approach has two essential logics underpinning it, which suggest two forms of communication:

* appeals to the self-interest of a community, individual, business or other organization, and/or to their sense of community obligation; or
* an assumption that there is a knowledge deficit (if people have the knowledge provided by an awareness campaign, the assumption goes, they will do what is thought to be appropriate by emergency management officials; although this assumption holds in some circumstances, there is little evidence for its general applicability).

Table 6.3 *Coercive, cooperative and exhortative policy designs*

	Coercive policy	Cooperative policy	Exhortation
Policy objective	Adherence to prescribed standards	Achievement of policy goals	Partial achievement of policy goals
Role of implementing authority	Regulatory agents: enforce rules or regulations prescribed by higher-level governments	Regulatory partners: develop and apply rules that are consistent with higher-level goals	Responsible authority: uses persuasion to achieve compliance
Emphasis of higher-level government policy	Prescribe regulatory actions and plans, along with a required process	Prescribe process and goals: specify planning considerations, along with performance standards	Specify desirable actions
Control of implementing authority	Monitoring for procedural compliance: enforcement and penalties for failing to meet deadlines or for not adhering to the prescribed process	Monitoring for substantive compliance: financial inducements to develop plans; advice; no penalties	Monitoring for compliance and targeting advice; no penalties; inducements may be possible
Assumptions about implementation	Commitment of implementing authority is a potential problem; need for uniform application of policies	Commitment is not a problem; local discretion is important in implementation	Awareness builds commitment; information helps capacity; expertise and material may support capacity
Implementation emphasis	Adherence to detailed policy prescriptions and regulatory standards Building 'calculated' commitment	Building capacity of local government to reach policy goals Enhancing 'normative' commitment	Changing attitudes to build strong commitment

| Potential problems | Weak monitoring of performance and unwillingness to use penalties | Gaps in local commitment and insufficient resources to build capacity Possibility of 'capture' | High level of non-compliance; may raise commitment without capacity |
| Ideological orientation | Central government can prescribe local ideology | Emphasis on performance and accountability means choice of ideology at the local level | People/local entities have responsibility for their risks |

Source: adapted from May and Handmer (1992)

In both forms of communication, it is assumed that the capacity to implement the policy exists or can be easily acquired, and the exhortation concentrates on building commitment. It is entirely voluntary, so it has the disadvantage that compliance would usually be partial, but generally has the great advantage of low costs for the responsible officials, and lesser risks of political or community backlash.

Cooperation

The cooperative approach to policy design attempts to make those at risk (or lower levels of government) partners in achieving emergency management or policy goals (see Table 6.3). It places the responsibility for risk management onto those at risk or their local governments or community institutions, and concentrates on enhancing their ability or capacity to reach these goals. Implicit are the assumptions that those at risk are committed to the same goals and that they will cooperate with higher level government. Emphasis is usually placed on regulatory or performance goals (e.g. public safety and decreased flood damage potential), rather than prescribed standards (e.g. prohibiting floodplain development), under the presumption that local governments or community members will devise the best means within their communities to reach such goals. Such local goal-setting is viewed as less politically confrontational and/or more effective because of local commitment and knowledge.

Typically, incentives are offered by higher levels of government for cooperation by lower levels, in contrast to the penalties used in coercive policy design. Among other things, incentives may be money, technical assistance or even immunity from legal liability (on this last point, see, for example, NSW, 2001, p30). Cash or technical advice for retrofitting buildings, making gardens more fire resistant, the installation of smoke alarms or the provision of a facilitator to help those at risk reach decisions on what to do are typical examples. A cooperative approach is inherently flexible and recognizes that the achievement of one goal involves trade-offs with other goals, such as economic development, and must have the cooperation of local government or other key entities. It has the ability to retreat in the face of strong opposition, while remaining ready to make progress as opportunities arise. Inevitably, this orientation requires increased use of negotiation and conflict resolution skills, which requires a framework within which negotiation can occur.

Potential difficulties with this approach are the need for adequate resources of funds and expertise to build capacity; the possibility that the flexibility may result in change that is incremental and too slow; that sectoral interests might 'capture' the process; the extended time period required to build trust and establish programmes; and lack of penalties to use against those who are recalcitrant.

Coercion

In a coercive approach, governments set out detailed regulatory standards and procedures to be implemented by local entities or those at risk in order to achieve policy goals. In effect, where local governments are involved, they may become an agent following specific instructions from above. Coercion comes from mechanisms for monitoring the actions of local entities and others required to implement the policy, and in the form of penalties for failure to comply. In Florida, for example, local jurisdictions can be, and are, fined for failure to comply with a coercive hazard management regime (May et al, 1996). The approach presumes conflicts between the various levels of government over goals, or over the means to meet these goals. It concentrates on building (or, rather, forcing) commitment instead of capacity.

Limitations with coercion stem from the need for adequate monitoring and penalties to force compliance, which often do not exist or are very difficult or costly to apply. One reason for this difficulty is the potential for a political backlash that may threaten the whole policy, as occurred in New South Wales, Australia (Handmer, 1986). In reality, strong opposition will often lead to negotiated solutions.

Mixed policy programmes

In practice, it is rare for any one of these three general classes of policy approach to be used in isolation. Policy programmes utilizing multiple approaches and instruments are common, if not always successful, in emergency management. For example, a flood preparedness strategy may include hard rules on land development, a cooperative, ongoing planning process, and public education campaigns backed up by mandatory evacuations in crisis periods. Mixed instrument packages fit with changes in thinking around policy and regulation generally, arguing for, and commenting on, a more flexible approach that includes self-regulation and incentive-based policy mechanisms as well as, or in place of, straight 'command' regulation (see Gunningham and Grabosky, 1999; Braithwaite and Drahos, 2000). Often, a hierarchy of instruments is advocated, starting with the 'softer' instruments of information provision and self-regulation, through to fallback 'harder' instruments, where necessary, to correct non-compliance. However, the life and property costs of disasters imply a quite different threshold between using persuasion and exercising authority in emergency situations, compared to many other policy domains. The critical question is whether the mixture is appropriate to the situation and whether the different components are implemented in a coordinated fashion. Three simple questions, if closely considered, will enhance the prospects of successful implementation:

1　What weighting is appropriate between the 'harder' and 'softer' components of the policy package, considering the scale and timing of the potential event and the political context?
2　In what sequence should different policy styles and instruments be developed and applied, taking into account the nature of the problem and the political and social context?
3　What are the implementation requirements for the different components (information, skills, institutional capacity, time, finance, etc.) and, importantly, are the different organizations to be involved in implementation capable of coordinated action?

Key to successful implementation of any policy response is an appropriate institutional system with sufficient capacity to handle complex policy tasks and whole-of-government and whole-of-society coordination, a matter taken up further in Chapter 8.

Implementation attributes

Where commitment is lacking, coercion may be needed to achieve results, although little will be achieved if those responsible for implementation lack the capacity to do so. Whatever approach to policy design is adopted, the attributes of capacity and commitment are required by those responsible for implementation.

Capacity

Although implementation capacity is required for all three approaches, the emphasis varies. As mentioned earlier, cooperative policy designs emphasize capacity-building, while more coercive approaches – and exhortation – tend to assume that the necessary capacity exists and concentrate on ensuring commitment. Capacity may be conceptualized as:

> ... the ability to anticipate and influence change; make informed, intelligent decisions about policy; develop programmes to implement policy; attract and absorb resources; manage resources; and evaluate current activities to guide future action. (Honadle, 1981)

In practical terms, capacity may refer to, among other things, possession of adequate funds and expertise, or the ability to obtain these through grants, technical assistance and training and development, including organizational development. It also refers to the ability to learn, to negotiate, to mobilize support for its objectives, and to take possession of an adequate legal framework. The funding aspect is often overplayed as information or human resources may be just as (if not more) critical, and organizations may lack the ability to absorb substantial increases in resources. Requirements for planning and the existence of plans have been found to enhance local capacity and to build constituencies (Burby and Dalton, 1994). One issue is whether capacity is weakened or strengthened by the commercialization of government activities, introducing complexity in information transactions and a greater number of players (e.g. consultancies and out-sourced firms) (Hood and Jackson, 1992). In summary, capable organizations are forward thinking, learning, adaptive, networked with other organizations, politically astute, and able to solve problems. And such organizations will have an adequately accepted mandate to undertake their function, whether that mandate is stated in law or based on more informal understanding.

Potential indicators of capacity by local government include:

- size relative to population;
- legal power or authority;
- process for implementation.

Potential indicators for both those at risk and local entities include:

- personal networks and access to technical expertise;
- availability of money; and
- adequacy of the information base.

Commitment

Local implementing authorities may have the capacity to implement emergency management programmes but see them as a low priority for a variety of reasons. They may believe that there is not a local problem, or they may be unwilling to cooperate because of perceived difficulties with the policy or with other organizations or individuals involved. For example, they may believe that they lack the necessary legal authority; be fully absorbed dealing with other local problems; be under pressure to allow development to proceed unheeded in, for instance, flood-prone areas; or have no support from their constituents. Maintaining commitment for emergency management-related policy is especially difficult during lengthy quiet periods – suggesting that attention to commitment cannot be ignored except when events are frequent and dramatic enough to maintain high levels of attention.

Lack of commitment is a serious problem that can undermine otherwise excellent policies and perhaps even lead to total failure. The cooperative-type policies tend to assume that commitment to the policy objectives exists. When it does not exist, performance will be poor. In contrast, the coercive approach assumes that commitment is lacking and works to create it. An obvious way of encouraging commitment is to make emergency management a legal requirement, with penalties for non-compliance, building what is known as *calculated commitment* (May et al, 1996). Commitment may also emerge through the professional standards or expectations placed on relevant staff, such as local government officials. It may seem appropriate that local priorities and risk perceptions should be respected. Unfortunately, the risk with this approach is that a major problem may evolve in the absence of appropriate hazard management if, for example, substantial unconstrained development occurs in hazardous areas.

Information targeted at government officials or the public may help to build commitment. Some people may use the information to lobby for emergency management action, thereby prompting political commitment. Another way of incorporating information is to draw it into a formal planning process, ensuring a greater level of formal recognition and likely a longer life span of relevance.

Potential measures of commitment by local governments include:

- commitment by elected officials;
- commitment by senior professional local staff;
- codification in plans and procedures;
- influence of emergency management staff.

Potential measures of commitment by those at risk and other local entities include:

- regular discourse with community institutions;
- legal requirements recognized and acted on;
- established local practices.

When local governments and local-scale community and private organizations lack commitment to higher-level policy objectives, a coercive approach produces better results, as measured by local effort and compliance with specified procedures (May et al, 1996). But where commitment already exists, a cooperative approach leads to results equal to or better than those achieved under coercion. In addition, it appears that cooperative policies may be superior in maintaining local government commitment, especially where processes that include stakeholders are used to spread and maintain shared understanding.

Conclusion

Selection of policy instruments should be guided by what will most likely achieve the desired results, but also by what is acceptable and what can be implemented – it is more important that policy instruments work well in practice than in theory. The benefits of hazard specific measures are usually evident in that they are about the detail of managing a particular risk in a particular place. But their costs and limitations are also clear. Generic measures that target vulnerability more broadly are often closely connected with community development and may therefore be assumed to be mainstream parts of a government's agenda. However, often they are not. All options should be considered and, if possible, used in concert since both are needed: the specific measures will often not work properly without the robust institutions and level of human development promised by more generic approaches. Any measure must take account of, and sit comfortably with, the 'universal' instruments of policy – economics, law, institutions and communication.

The three policy styles of coercion, cooperation and exhortation that are set out here all require a commitment to implementation and the capacity to do so. These three styles are one construction of the range of policy choices. Other constructions are possible; but the key challenge remains to maintain a wide menu of policy instruments and to choose according to the challenges faced, rather than rely on unthinking predisposition.

7

Not Forgetting: Monitoring, Evaluation and Learning

It may seem commonsense to emphasize the importance of learning from experience in order to improve future policy responses and institutional capacities. Surely this is normal practice? Ideally, as policies are implemented, routines for capturing the necessary data are put in place, the effectiveness of policy interventions are monitored, and formal evaluations feed into the redesign of polices. However, in the emergencies area and elsewhere in public policy, careful harvesting of insights from past and current experience and purposeful application of the knowledge thus gained to adapt and improve capacities are too often not evident. This chapter identifies key issues that, if addressed, will enable policy learning and improvement, allowing for the design and maintenance of adaptive policy processes and institutional settings. It goes beyond the more familiar and well-documented practice of monitoring and evaluation, considering the nature of policy learning, conducive institutional characteristics, basic forms of information and their routine capture, and the development of human capacities.

The point of 'not forgetting' is to learn and improve. The usual language describing this activity is *monitoring and evaluation* (M&E), representing an ever-growing enterprise in government and associated consultancies, and targeted at operational project and programme evaluation. Consequently, our coverage of M&E is a brief summary later in this chapter, with most space devoted to the broader concept of *policy learning*, since this is more relevant to the themes of this book.

Uncertainty, time and learning

Emergencies and disasters, as a policy domain, have a number of characteristics that make policy learning at once crucially needed and highly difficult. Drawing on Chapters 1 and 2, it is worth revisiting selected attributes of policy problems in the domain in terms of how they shape the challenge of monitoring, evaluation and learning:

- *Extended and multiple scales of time and space*, where knowledge and memory of events may span many years, even generations, and cross political and administrative boundaries. This complicates understanding of, preparedness for and response to disasters by spreading roles and information across time and space, and making cross-event and cross-context transfer of lessons difficult.

- *Pervasive uncertainty* surrounding the causes and magnitude of possible events, and vulnerabilities and capacities under different disaster scenarios. Importantly, no matter how good the knowledge base and the understanding of vulnerabilities and capacities, the existence of inevitable residual uncertainty and the possibility of surprise throw doubt on the efficacy of the hardest-won lessons.
- Imperatives for wide *community participation* in management and policy. Positively, this broader engagement (see Chapter 4) widens the catchment of experience and knowledge available to inform learning. However, the more inclusive and broad the membership of the policy community, the more challenging policy learning becomes: communication, organization, and development of mutual understanding among a diversity of actors with a diversity of values, interests, information-processing capacities and organizational strengths.
- The high and often urgent '*stakes*' in disaster situations – lives lost, livelihoods ruined and environments degraded – are a strong argument for sophisticated policy learning. But combined with uncertainty in various forms, they also make lesson-drawing a complicated task, more contested and politically sensitive, and thus a more hazardous activity for the policy analyst. In a professional and organizational sense, close attention to the performance of policy and institutional settings involves risks to individuals, agencies and political leaders, especially at times when attribution of blame is sought in post-disaster debates. The lulls of attention and resources between disasters can be difficult times in which to maintain interest.
- Vulnerability to disasters is determined by factors located deep in social and economic situations *(indirect or systemic causes)* – patterns of settlement, resource dependency, economic condition, livelihood security, infrastructure and health systems – as well as more immediate causes such as building quality. Analysis of how well policy and institutional measures attend to these causes and to prescriptions is complicated and difficult, but is needed if vulnerability is to be reduced.
- Emergencies and disasters entail *cross-sectoral and whole-of-government* responsibilities and implications. While this is reasonably well accepted in more immediate emergency planning and response, it is less apparent in terms of integrated policy and institutional settings to ensure that pre-event and ongoing disaster policy brings together different parts of government and society. The generation of relevant information and policy lessons across sectors and portfolios is necessarily harder than in policy domains where responsibilities are more narrowly contained.

Despite these challenges, emergency management probably learns from experience more than most professional fields: perhaps only health and medicine puts as much effort and thought into lesson-drawing from experience. This is not surprising since both share the attributes of high stakes, political and moral imperatives and sensitivities, and complex systems with multiple cause–effect linkages. Emergency management agencies and individuals review events, debrief staff and communities, communicate lessons and warnings, and take accreditation procedures and competency standards built on accrued experience very seriously. They are held routinely accountable and are closely evaluated for their performance by coronial courts, commissions of inquiries and the like, as well as in the larger 'court' of public and political opinion. Nevertheless, most of this information-gathering and learning focuses on preparedness for likely or known disaster events, and on related and more immediate response and recovery capacities. The emphasis in this book is on the policy and institutional capacities within which operational emergency management operates and is either enabled or constrained. There is less formalized evaluation of these settings, and the ways in which this can be more clearly thought about is the focus of this section.

Warning signs of impending disaster are very often ignored for a wide range of reasons clearly set out by authors such as Turner (1978); and Turner and Pidgeon (1997) and Perrow (1984), as well as others who work on risk management in a corporate environment (e.g. Hopkins, 2005) and on many post-disaster public inquiries. It is frequently the case that it is very difficult for indicators, whether for a dam collapse, major industrial or transportation accident or other incident, to become part of emergency decision-making that leads to action. Such problems and failure to learn arise from organizational attributes and cultures that inhibit problem acknowledgment, learning and even minor change. They also generally arise because of near-term economic imperatives in consideration of emergency management, most readily seen in the development of areas prone to flooding, wildfire, landslide and so on. Often, the people concerned may be aware of the risks but may feel that they have no option, such as those crowded around the Union Carbide plant in Bhopal.

The case of a 1966 mining spoil heap collapse in Aberfan, south Wales, illustrates some of the organizational issues. The problems were well known in the village and had been brought to the attention of authorities on several occasions through different channels. No action was taken and the tip collapsed onto the village school, killing 144 people, including many of the area's school children. The post-disaster inquiry condemned the British Coal Board for, among other, things ignoring warnings well before the disaster (McLean and Johnes, 2000). Following the Aberfan disaster, US authorities examined similar sites across the US. One such site was a tailings dam at Buffalo Creek, West Virginia. The local coal industry had a long history of safety-related problems; but even though the risks were clear, activities continued as normal. On 26 February 1972, the tailings dam collapsed, eliminating villages, killing 125, injuring over 1000 and making 4000 homeless (Erikson, 1976, 1979).

One test for whether information from monitoring and warnings – formal or informal – is likely to be useful is whether information on near-misses comes to the attention of decision-makers in real time. As the human-made contributing factors to emergencies and disasters are scattered across portfolios, sectors and places (spatial planning, transport, chemical approvals, engineering standards, and many more), emergency managers can hardly be expected to gather information from across government, society and industry. The whole-of-government nature of comprehensive disaster policy is emphasized.

If policy and institutional learning is rarer than it should be – and the disasters field is not alone in facing this situation – then the first step in advancing the endeavour should be a clarification of what such learning is, why it is pursued and by whom.

Policy and institutional learning: Purposes and forms

It is obvious that policy learning is a good thing, but less obvious that it occurs frequently or effectively. Furthermore, what it precisely entails is unclear.[1] On the first of these, it is widely suggested that deliberate, well-structured and *effective learning is not common in public policy*. Although learning does occur, it is generally in a haphazard and less than optimally effective manner. It is worth considering why, and some obvious reasons can be proposed. The first is simply that evaluation of policy experiences and distillation of lessons requires time and resources, and these are often not in abundant supply in either government or in interested NGOs. Second, skills and experience in such policy analysis may not be available or may be imperfect. Third, it may not be thought politically wise to engage in evaluation of experience lest failure be described and advertised, or key individuals and groups may be protective of their expertise and discourage scrutiny. Fourth, the necessary information regarding policy and institutional performance may not be available: it may not have been identified as relevant and routinely collected, or it may have been difficult to obtain. Fifth, there may not be an authority or organization with sufficient mandate or capacity to drive a process of review, evaluation and lesson-drawing. Finally, the brief periods of post-event interest so common in emergencies and disasters may be insufficient to engage adequate interest and resources in evaluation and learning. Given the difficult attributes of policy problems in disasters, some of these issues can be expected to be particularly acute. These issues are explored here and in Chapter 8.

A further reason is that the varying purposes and forms of learning are not always clearly conceptualized, understood and implemented in appropriate ways. We turn to that now. The first basic principle is that *effective policy learning rarely entails mimicry*, but rather the accessing of relevant lessons and insights, carefully distilled and applied. The unthinking transfer of what appeared successful elsewhere or before is unlikely to be appropriate: contexts differ too much. Another basic principle is that useful insights can come from all sorts of experiences, whether positive or negative. In fact, complete policy success is as rare as total failure, and in the majority of disaster experiences, along the continuum between success and failure there exist myriad possibilities for lesson-drawing (the issue of identifying appropriate resolutions for learning is discussed below).

But most important for policy learning is the embedding of responsibilities, procedures and information streams within policy formulation and implementation stages, and not as an afterthought. Policy goals, the policy instruments being used, the legal responsibilities for aspects of implementation, and administrative structures used – all of these determine why, how and by who policy monitoring and evaluation can and will be undertaken. Evaluation as afterthought, prompted by a rediscovered clause stating that 'this policy will be reviewed in X years time' will generally encounter an absence of data, unclear and immeasurable goals, and no clear responsibility for evaluation. As a result, proper understanding of success and failure will not be possible and opportunities for improvement will be missed.

Monitoring and evaluation of policy and institutional settings may be thought of as having four possible outcomes, depending on the degree to which policy goals are attained:

1 *cessation* of a policy intervention, with policy goals achieved;
2 *continuation* of a policy intervention or institutional/organizational structure, with goals approached satisfactorily but not yet attained;
3 *revision* of a policy and/or institutional settings in light of poor performance and demonstrable low likelihood of achieving the goals of the whole programme or setting, or of parts thereof, whether radically or more moderately;
4 *redefinition* of the policy problem in light of new information and understanding, involving significant redesign of policy interventions.

It is important to recognize that different individuals, interests and organizations will have quite different reasons for wishing to learn from policy experiments, and that, occasionally, these multiple reasons will invite collaboration and joint learning, whereas at other times there may be clear conflict (e.g. constructive lesson-drawing versus blame attribution). Table 7.1 identifies some basic differences in the forms and purposes of policy learning.

It is apparent from Table 7.1 that the intent of an exercise in policy learning can vary significantly in terms of who undertakes it, what the subject is, forms of information and analysis that might be used, and what insights might arise from it. Frequently, more than one of the four forms of learning listed in Table 7.1 will be pursued at one time, whether by a single actor or by several in concert. In such cases, clarity of purpose is necessary, a judgement which should also include an explanation of why other forms of learning (and, thus, information) are not being pursued. As with the principle of exclusion through inclusive design described in Chapter 4, a decision to evaluate in a particular way may involve an implicit decision not to evaluate other things.

An important distinction exists between forms 1 and 2 (instrumental and government), which operate *within* existing problem definition and social and policy goals, and forms 3 and 4 (social and political), which allow and, indeed, intend to reconsider and possibly reframe policy and/or social problems and goals. Thus, the implications of social and political learning for future policy styles and for institutional arrangements may be profound, whereas instrumental and government learning are simply about how to perform better. Social learning returns us to stages 1 and 2 in Figure 3.2 in Chapter 3 (problem and policy framing), whereas instrumental and government learning involve a reiteration of stage 3 (policy design and implementation).

Referring to Table 2.1 in Chapter 2 – key components of the governing state – there are numerous locations of potential policy learning, with different actors playing sometimes distinct and sometimes joint roles in generating, receiving and acting on information. These include government agencies, NGOs, the courts, regulatory bodies, research organizations and informal community institutions, and within these there is, again, considerable variation in motivation, capacity and mandate.

Table 7.1 *Forms and purposes of policy learning*

Form	What is learned?	Who learns?	Intended result
1 Instrumental learning	How policy instruments and implementation procedures have performed relative to stated goals	Core members of relevant policy network, especially those governmental officials and close non-government partners responsible for policy implementation *Example:* fire brigade captains	Redesign of existing or better design of future policy instrument and detailed implementation procedures *Example:* household receptiveness to issued fire safety guideline brochures
2 Government learning	How administrative structures and processes have contributed to or limited policy implementation	Members of the policy network, especially senior government officials and key stakeholders accountable for design and maintenance of policy process *Example:* ambulance, health and rescue service senior staff	Redesign of existing or better design of future administrative structures and processes *Example:* coordinated emergency warning systems involving two levels of government and multiples agencies
3 Social learning	The relevance and usefulness of policies and policy and social goals	The broader policy community, including both more and less closely engaged actors within and outside government *Example:* regional planning organization, including local government, industry and community representatives	Reframed problems and goals via altered understanding of cause–effect understanding or social preferences *Example:* shift from top-down emergency preparedness to community resilience approach

| 4 Political learning | How to engage effectively with and influence political and policy processes | Actors wishing to enhance ability to change policy agendas and outcomes or to defend and maintain existing ones. *Example:* agricultural lobby groups seeking to shift policy on fuel-reduction burning on state land | Changes in problem definition, policy goals, membership of the policy network and power of particular groups *Example:* use of post-event political opportunities to gain interest group membership of key committee |

Source: adapted from Bennett and Howlett (1992), May (1992) and Connor and Dovers (2004)

The shift in emergency management and in policy and institutional theory and practice, more broadly, towards networked or more inclusive modes of operation (see Chapter 4) further extends the responsibility of policy learning. So does the whole-of-government and whole-of-society nature of emergencies and disasters. The most apparent and obvious locations of policy learning, and the monitoring and evaluation that informs it, are the emergency services organizations that are directly responsible (fire, ambulance, health services, emergency management, search and rescue, and so on) and the policy agencies which oversee these. Yet, these are only some of the locations of policy learning in the institutional landscape. With wildfire, for example, local brigades, their central offices and local fire-prone communities have a clear role in instrumental policy learning. But local institutions (schools, churches, community service groups and major employers) also play a strong role in preparedness, response and recovery, as well as local government. Executive government oversees and directs much of the relevant policy and generally is the initiator of major reviews. In terms of reducing vulnerability through managing the landscape in which fire occurs, planners, architects, construction materials researchers, public health agencies, vegetation scientists, meteorological bureaus, farmer organizations, national parks services, forestry agencies and more will – or at least should – be concerned with various forms of policy learning.

This diffuse spread of interests and responsibilities creates challenges in coordination and information transfer across government and across parts of the community. A particular issue comprises the optimal forms of evaluation to capture the spread of players and to deal with both ongoing operational issues (instrumental) and other forms of learning (government and social). We will ignore, for the moment, the role of political learning on the basis that proper attention paid to government and social learning will provide opportunities for such tactical learning by advocates, and that inclusive policy processes and institutions will assist in managing advocacy in a constructive, rather than destructive or biased, manner.

Instrumental learning

Instrumental learning for normal emergency management operational matters is well established, and is directed at ensuring effectiveness and efficiency for the full range of normal activities. In practice, the distinction between these approaches and those generally seen as more about change may not be clear cut since basic training can be used to inculcate change. Training is the universal approach, providing the skills needed by emergency managers. Although it is now increasingly based on formal achievement of 'competencies', much is delivered informally through experienced colleagues and is learned through practice. In addition to formal and informal training via instructors, debriefs usually follow significant events. Those participating in a debrief may have been at the event in question, or learning may occur from experiences elsewhere.

Occasionally, however, the skills acquired cannot be applied properly. Common reasons for this include the absence of a clear mission or the fact that resources, including staff, may be used for other purposes within the agency. Organizational culture may block application because of the inertia of past, inappropriate practices, constant internal change or the absence of planning for the non-routine. The organization may be powerless or treated as irrelevant by other agencies and those at risk. Wasteful inter-organizational competition may also prevent emergency management from achieving its aims.

Training, debriefs and other such measures all presuppose the existence of appropriate processes. This is now frequently organized through state or national focal points, such as the Emergency Management Australia Institute or the US Federal Emergency Management Authority Institute at Emmitsburg, as well as local government meetings and fora. Tertiary-education institutions also play an important role, as do some professional associations, such as the US State Floodplain Managers Association and various industry and fire and emergency service groups. The International Committee on Large Dams (ICOLD) and its national equivalents were established during the 1930s as professional associations that have since been instrumental in developing safety standards for large dams. While we mention such groups in the context of learning and improvement, other groups can also reinforce tradition and resist improvement, or change in ways that enhance their finances or political profile, rather than augment safety and emergency management imperatives. Processes can, by themselves, encourage learning and change through exposure to different perspectives – multi-agency/organizational processes dedicated to debate and negotiation, such as inter-agency committees, can do this. One major driver of change in many countries, across all hazards, is public inquiry and associated legal processes, which can force change by demanding that it is needed to satisfy legal requirements, or through top-down political direction resulting from media pressure.

Opportunities for change

Particular times when policy change is rendered more likely by events and conditions are referred to as *policy windows* (Kingdon, 1984; Howlett, 1998). It is widely accepted that significant opportunities for reflection on policy and for policy change, or for more profound institutional change, arise especially immediately after a significant disaster event when human, environmental or economic losses are experienced. These are unpredictable policy windows. Such opportunities may be defined by considered reflection on the adequacy of preparation and response (see below), or by more immediate public outrage, or a combination of both. While these opportunities for policy learning are a positive phenomenon, they carry dangers. They are, by definition, unpredictable, often short lived and can be highly political, inviting 'garbage can'-style responses (see Chapter 2) in the absence of a solid body of information and understanding built up over time. A reactive intent of 'getting things back to normal' in such situations can overshadow consideration of more proactive strategies for reducing vulnerability in more long-lasting and preventative ways.

Other policy windows are more predictable, and policy actors (whether inside or outside government) can plan for such windows of opportunity and utilize them to inform policy learning. These opportunities include elections, changes of govern-ment, the mandated review period for a policy programme, budget cycles and the seasonal onset of some hazards (such as wildfire or cyclone season, the monsoon and mosquito-borne diseases, winter storms and snowmelt flooding).

Nevertheless, the nature of disasters is that unpredictable policy windows will arise, and suitable styles of evaluation can at least be understood and made ready for the eventuality. Four quite separate purposes of post-event reviews can be defined. First, operational-level reviews of technical and organizational performance are commonplace and inform future practices, such as evacuation procedures, warning systems and equipment adequacy. Second, reviews of the policy and institutional settings, often conflated with operational reviews, seek to analyse the appropri-ateness of inter-agency links, lines of command and so on. Third, reviews of the understanding of hazard type and frequency may be necessary, especially follow-ing an unexpected or unexpectedly large event. Fourth are investigations aimed at defining responsibility, blame and possible liability for lapses in performance and subsequent losses. Although related, these four purposes of post-event reviews are quite different in terms of the burdens of proof, evidence and information, the requisite skills of those involved, who participates, the authority under which they operate, and the formality of the process. Confusion between different purposes may not help policy learning. Institutional settings to enable such reviews are discussed in Chapter 8.

Learning from elsewhere

Earlier, various reasons were proposed for a lack of policy learning. Thus far we have considered learning within a reasonably tightly defined organizational or professional domain, such as the set of connected organizations concerned with emergencies in a given jurisdiction. Another reason for a lack of learning about better possible policy and institutional settings is a shortage of case studies: of sufficiently relevant information that can be examined and mined for insights. Given the immense variety of the types and contexts of disasters and their sporadic occurrence, it may be that policy lessons need to be sought from other jurisdictions or other policy sectors.

The attributes that define emergencies and disasters as policy and institutional problems – uncertainty, variable time scales, cross-sectoral impact, etc. – are shared by other policy and management domains, such as natural resource management, community development focused on resilience or public health. Some of the policy sectors already have relationships with emergency agencies, at least in an occasional functional sense, if not in joint policy analysis. The potential for information exchange and joint analysis to inform policy and institutional learning as opposed to operational collaboration is arguably under-developed. For example, risk communication strategies or mechanisms to maintain agency readiness for unpredictable threats are difficult challenges that confront not only emergency managers.

The other means of expanding the catchment of information, ideas and possible strategies is through other areas and jurisdictions. Again, the point of such comparative policy analysis is not to copy what has been done elsewhere, but to learn from it. The basis of lesson-drawing from other jurisdictions should be clear for reasons of efficiency (not to waste effort seeking insights fruitlessly) and of effectiveness (gaining usable insights). Two ways of ensuring such clarity are to consider, first, the basis of comparison or contrast, and, second, the level in the hierarchy of management, policy and institutions to which the lessons are relevant. On the first of these, the basis of comparison and/or contrast may include similarities in:

- hazard types (e.g. flash floods, toxic chemical release or earthquakes) or context of hazard (e.g. low-lying tropical coasts, remote river valley farming, the occurrence of informal peri-urban settlements, abandoned dams, or hazardous industries);
- socio-economic or cultural contexts, such as household structure, stages of development, demographic character, social structure, communication infrastructure, dominant industries or degree of urbanization;
- political and legal systems and, thus, general policy opportunities and constraints (e.g. federal systems or highly autonomous local authorities);
- policy styles or instruments, or delivery and implementation systems (e.g. reliance on volunteerism or market mechanisms, or coercive versus cooperative policy approaches).

None of the above, or other bases of comparison, are better or worse as a filter for identifying useful information and examples than others, nor are they mutually exclusive. In some ways, the exercise of justifying the basis for comparison is as much a case of guarding against inappropriate foci for analysis and lesson-drawing as it is for identifying the optimal. The second consideration is the level in the institutional system where the lessons or insights being pursued are relevant. We can identify four – again, not mutually exclusive, but quite different as sources of insight and potentially transferable information and ideas:

1 *general policy styles and institutional options*, such as another jurisdiction that has experimented with a different overall approach (e.g. a volunteer-based rather than central agency-driven response capacity, or collaborative rather than coercive policy styles);
2 examples at the level of *policy programme or organizational model*, with the intent

or possibility of transferring the 'blueprint' from one context to another (e.g. a risk management framework to replace or supplement existing prescriptive standards);

3   *detailed subcomponents* of policy programmes and organizational models, such as communication strategies within a programme, aspects of regulatory design or cross-agency coordination plans;

4   *operational and technological options and elements*, less dependent than the above on contextual variation (although it will still be important), including 'hardware' (such as communication devices or fire-suppressant delivery systems) or 'software' (such as computer programmes or training modules).

As with the bases for comparison, the question is not which of these is best, but which is most appropriate or important to the individual or group seeking ideas. The last – technological and operational options – is normal practice and routinely undertaken without too much risk of adopting seriously flawed ideas (assuming that resourcing and maintenance capacities are considered). The second level – transfer of policy or organizational 'blueprints' – is unlikely to be wise in anything but *very* similar social, political and economic contexts, such as across provincial administrations in a federal system (and even then should be conducted with care). The most profitable levels of comparative policy analysis and, thus, policy learning, we believe, are more likely to be either the first or third levels: general policy ideas or detailed subcomponents of policy programmes and organizational designs.

In policy learning, it may be that it is easier to transfer negative lessons (i.e. do not let this happen; do not try this!) than it is to transfer positive ones (i.e. do it the recommended way) since the warning is often easier to adapt to a different context than an encouraging model, even though both demand careful analysis of what features of the policy or institutional intervention contributed to relative success or failure.

Reflecting on the examples set out in Chapter 1, Hurricane Katrina and its aftermath in New Orleans have generated a modest industry analysing the problems and causes, and advising others everywhere, even though direct relevance of this material is probably very limited (Handmer, 2006; see Box 1.1). In contrast, response to the Indian Ocean tsunami contains many successes that are arguably transferable at least in the context of a complex unbounded event, but have received relatively little attention (see Box 1.3).

More generic examples are provided by risk and modern communication technology. Risk-based approaches appear to have universal application – and they are being implemented everywhere, often with little attention to local context. But the approach has its limits (see Chapter 5) and can be harnessed to promote activities that may cause low probability problems for emergency management. In poorer areas, a risk-based approach could help to prioritize anticipated problems (e.g. levees for flooding), but should not deflect attention from improving resilience as part of development (e.g. access to credit).

Modern technology provides positive examples of learning and offers much promise. But equipment with expensive ongoing costs (e.g. volcanic monitoring dependent on satellite phones or specialist expertise for maintenance) is unlikely to continue functioning in areas where the funds or expertise are unavailable – a case of matching technology with context and capacity. At the other end of the warning system, modern information and communication technologies such as the internet and mobile phone have been enthusiastically adopted by people almost everywhere. Interesting differences in usage emerge, however: in the US, text messaging is less common, while in most of the world it is one of the most popular ways of communicating, with many private companies offering text warning services directly to the public. Here it is a case of emergency management agencies, rather than those at risk, needing to learn how best to utilize the technologies.

Basic information capture

In virtually any sector or portfolio, policy learning across events and circumstances will require ongoing data capture, analysis and dissemination to provide descriptions and understanding of basic processes and entities. Information richness and sensitivity comprise a fundamental attribute of an effective and adaptable policy and institutional system (see Chapter 3). In some policy areas, such basic information capture is well resourced and widely apparent, such as in finance, criminology and population censuses. Other policy sectors may not be as well serviced with information. In emergencies and disasters, where the focus of public and political attention is likely to be during and immediately after events of uncertain timing and often long periods of 'inactivity', there is a real danger of data capture being anything but routine, with short, intensive bursts of information-gathering punctuating longer periods of turpitude and amnesia. The disasters arena is particularly difficult as the requisite information and understanding must cover and enable comprehension of tightly interconnected natural and human systems defined by variables often outside our control, and which interact in vastly different ways depending on the context.

Policy learning and more operational-level monitoring and evaluation (see below), all of which seek to teach us to do things better, cannot be achieved without quality information inputs. Required areas of information can be defined according to four general categories, each of which will inform policy learning but also entail quite different forms of information and responsibilities for (and methods of) information-gathering:

1 *Biophysical* data and models of natural systems and variables that contribute to disasters, including climate, hydrological regimes and coastal terrain studies. In wealthy countries, natural systems are well monitored, albeit often not in a way that connects well with strategic disaster planning. Most jurisdictions have their monitoring agencies and there are also monitoring organizations that are global or globally connected (e.g. the US Geological Survey, national meteorological and seismological offices, or the Intergovernmental Panel on Climate Change). Contamination and industrial risks are less well monitored. In many poorer countries, monitoring of any type is limited.
2 *Socio-economic* determinants of vulnerability to disasters, including demographic

profile, education and literacy levels, security of livelihood, access to policy and decision-making processes, and health status. In most jurisdictions there is no monitoring of these factors specifically for disaster vulnerability. Only in particularly disaster-prone places are these factors considered in a systematic way. Major NGOs such as the Red Cross/Red Crescent, United Nations agencies such as the United Nations Children's Fund (UNICEF) and some aid agencies are active in these places.

3　The *capacity of response-and-recovery systems*, such as backup communications, the availability of health services, transport infrastructure, and local commerce for employment and retail distribution. These are all crucial features.

4　*Policy-related information*, such as the number of trained operatives, penetration of communication materials, expenditure of funds or the functioning of interdepartmental committees. There are many good examples at this level, although the existence of interdepartmental committees does not, by itself, indicate that they achieve their aims.

The biggest challenge is not determining what information is required (although this may not be a trivial exercise), but rather embedding responsibilities and mandates for information capture and delivery within the policy and institutional system, especially in a manner that ensures the ongoing maintenance of information flows. Two strategies to ensure such longevity in attention and effort can be noted. The first is to codify such information responsibilities in statutory mandates or at least in formal policy statements, such as intergovernmental agreements. The second is to allow wide participation in policy processes that design information systems in order to spread more widely knowledge of who is expected to do what – it is difficult not to undertake a publicly recognized duty and role.

Evaluation: The precondition for learning

Monitoring and evaluation (M&E) has become a basic function in public administration and in many parts of the private sector, and is well described elsewhere (see Patton, 2002; Wholey et al, 2004; the journals *Evaluation Practice* and *American Journal of Evaluation*). The focus in this book on policy learning and purposeful institutional change, and on the peculiar aspects of emergencies and disasters as a policy domain, suggest that the broader, rather than practical, issues of M&E are the most critical – that is, the connection between 'hands-on' evaluation and the policy and institutional system. From the framework identified in Figure 3.2 in Chapter 3, we can recall the broad attributes of adaptive policy processes and institutional settings:

- *purposefulness* consistent with widely understood problem statements and goals;
- *persistence*, with sufficient longevity in efforts to learn and adapt;
- *information richness and sensitivity*, involving not only the necessity for quality information, but also the wide accessibility of this information;

- *inclusiveness*, allowing for participation by stakeholders and the reconciliation of multiple values and perspectives;
- *flexibility*, so that purposefulness and persistence do not atrophy into rigidity and an inability to learn and adapt.

These institutional attributes will be further addressed in Chapter 8; but here we can consider how approaches to M&E can be more, rather than less, supportive of them in two ways: the characteristics of monitoring-related elements of the policy process and clarity over the purpose of evaluation. On the first of these, monitoring and subsequent evaluation will not be optimally effective without the following characteristics:

- *Explicit recognition of uncertainty* and, thus, of the necessarily contingent and experimental nature of policy and institutional responses. Without such explicit recognition of uncertainty, it is unlikely that the policy community will be prompted to establish procedures for critical reflection or procure the necessary information to enable this. While mounting policy interventions in the hypothesis-testing manner of adaptive management (Holling, 1978) may be difficult in a strict sense, the open recognition that an experiment is, indeed, being undertaken – as with a public awareness campaign, or the provision of incentives for household or business preparedness – demands greater clarity of what is known and unknown, and of predicted and speculated cause–effect links between policy problems, goals and responses.
- *Measurable policy goals*, if not in a quantified sense, then at least in a qualitative manner that is amenable to eventual evaluation of relative success and/or failure. Such goals may define an intended *process* or a desired *outcome* (or both), and, in general, will entail overarching goals and a hierarchy of component goals for different aspects of the policy problem and programme. Measures might include reducing the value of assets or activities exposed to various hazards and the vulnerability of these assets; measures of warning system performance; favourable cost–benefit ratios; or improved household awareness and preparedness.
- *Basic routine data capture*, designed within the policy programme and linked to policy goals and key variables affecting their attainment, with clearly defined responsibilities for gathering and maintaining information streams. Basic data include descriptions of baseline conditions at the time of implementation, without which relative change following the policy intervention will be difficult to assess. Disaster datasets are often of a good quality when they cover physical phenomena such as flood depths, earthquake frequency, cyclone/hurricane/typhoon strength, and major transport accidents. But in relation to our interest in vulnerability, damage and resilience, there are few consistent and reliable datasets. Most contain inconsistent material of unknown quality – which reinforces the importance of metadata: information about the data in terms of quality, accuracy, fitness for purpose, etc. The exceptions, such as quality datasets held by some insurers and some national agencies, may be severely limited in scope and accessibility.
- *Coordination of roles* and activities across agencies and non-governmental groups,

given that disasters will typically involve actions across governmental and social sectors. For effective M&E, this will often involve the participation of agencies and players for whom the provision of critical information is their only substantial engagement in disasters policy (e.g. a statistical agency for demographic and settlement data or a manufacturing sector for sales of fire-retardant building materials). It will also entail the empowerment and coordination of informal community organizations and those with few financial or administrative resources.

- *A clear mandate for M&E activities.* Although coordinated, multiple inputs will usually be required; coordination requires some degree of centralized responsibility and authority for ongoing information-gathering, dissemination and formal review processes. Finance departments or associated agencies often fulfil a general policy monitoring role, including disaster policy and programmes (e.g. the US General Accounting Office). In some jurisdictions, there are agencies tasked with developing performance indicators for all government activities, such as the Australian Productivity Commission. More usually, monitoring is undertaken by agencies or groups with mandates for particular hazards or risks, while evaluation is more *ad hoc* and is often undertaken by consultants.
- *Information made widely available* to all stakeholders relevant to the policy problem and response. This is necessary to ensure understanding and engagement, and to maintain trust between policy actors, as well as for the more traditional reasons of public accountability.[2] Information availability is a continuous issue for emergency managers. It is needed during and after a disaster for response and recovery, and is required in advance for all types of planning and awareness. The internet is rapidly becoming the tool for universal access to disaster information (e.g. the UK's Environment Agency's website provides flood zones marked on street maps of the whole country).

In terms of the purpose of evaluation (and, thus, forms of evaluation processes and methods, and the information demands that they define), we can identify five purposes of evaluation (adapted from Howlett and Ramesh, 2003):

1 *Process evaluation* examines specific projects and programmes with a view to generating insights into how to improve policy processes and organizational structures.
2 *Efficiency evaluation* focuses on the expenditure of resources and whether policy outcomes could have been achieved at lower cost.
3 *Effort evaluation* also deals with questions of efficiency, but looks particularly at the quality and adequacy of inputs to policy implementation (finance, time, expertise, administrative resources, etc.).

   The three approaches above all deal with key inputs, and form the basis of most contemporary 'performance indicators' for emergency management agencies. This may reflect the availability and ease of comparability of the data, rather than the data's inherent importance for emergency management. This is not to understate the importance of budgets and value for money.
4 *Performance evaluation* investigates the outcomes of a policy intervention irrespective of achievement of policy goals.

5   *Effectiveness evaluation* assesses an intervention in terms of the stated policy goals.

These last two approaches are understandably quite common for disaster management given the goals to protect lives, livelihoods and property, and the high profile of failures. Agencies typically assess their warnings against technical criteria, but less commonly against broad goals such as community safety, although a programme logic approach is being used by the Australian Bushfire Cooperative Research Centre to evaluate community safety programmes. Commerce is also active in this arena, purveying products claiming to help fulfil emergency management objectives. Defining policy goals and objectives in ways that are measurable often creates major challenges. 'Improved community safety' may be universally agreed on as a goal, but is subject to many interpretations and is insufficient as a target for evaluation. Less apparent agendas cannot be ignored either: rapid response and visibility may be more important for the organization's profile and, thus, ongoing budget allocation than more substantive outputs.

All of these purposes are equally valid and may well be combined in an evaluation process; but, as with participation in Chapter 4, different actors will have different purposes and expectations. Some actors may only be concerned with the expenditure of public resources, others with the achievement of policy goals without any concern for expense, others with the inclusiveness of the policy process, and so on. These agendas need to be clearly defined in order to avoid confusion and so that appropriate information and methods are employed.

The particular attributes of the disasters domain suggests that the goal of preventing human, environmental and economic losses would always be paramount – but this is not necessarily the case. Questions of process, of financial efficiency, of administrative accountability – these are inevitable concerns and are important especially in terms of long-term processes and trust. Ideally, process and outcome-oriented evaluations can be designed in a coordinated fashion where different agendas are pursued constructively in the interests of policy learning.

Thus far, our focus has been on the monitoring and evaluation of specific policy and institutional responses. Underpinning capacities to undertake such M&Es, and even more so the ability to engage in policy learning, are the human skills and knowledge in the emergencies and disasters domain. This is very much influenced by research and education – what we can achieve is often determined by the appropriateness of the human resources and intelligence at our disposal.

Research and education

In the world of disasters and emergencies, there is a well-supported research tradition of studying geophysical phenomena. The picture is broadly similar for most industrial hazards, contaminants, transportation and other technological risks. Research is ongoing as part of science's function to generate an understanding of the natural world and to support the development of technology, and because these hazards are themselves dynamic. There is also much relevant research output from sociology, psychology, human geography, development studies, global change, economics, architecture and similar areas – although much less than from the physical sciences. Probably because much research in emergencies and disasters is strongly problem led, there are good examples of integrative research – research which includes a range of dimensions, including the geophysical or technological hazard, and the impacts on people, livelihoods and economies.

Critically under-researched areas include the areas of policy and institutions, and the broad domain of complex unbounded problems. Aspects of non-routine problems are also often poorly served. This is not surprising since emergency management has attracted funds and profiles primarily through its immediate and obvious actions, rather than its long-term risk reduction activities, and certainly not its broader role in vulnerability reduction. While politically very attractive when things go well, there is a tendency to search for the blameworthy for even minor errors. This often makes engagement with policy and politics problematic for researchers who seek to analyse the cause and effect of such errors. One challenge for all research is the tendency now for much work to be conducted under commercial agreements where the outcomes are not in the public domain and are therefore unavailable to many of those who need them. Similar comments can be made concerning counter-terrorism or security research. This issue is becoming widespread, affecting many government and university research groups as they link closely with the private sector or work in counter-terrorism.

Formal education and training are well documented, materials are readily available, and the training can be (and often is) delivered through tertiary colleges and by emergency management agencies themselves. Courses and qualifications up to Masters and PhD level are available in many countries. There is some tension between academic qualifications and the practical skills that are vital in multi-sectoral planning and preparation, as well as in response. Practical skills alone may be of limited value in strategic planning and institutional design. All are needed. The major potential gap is not in academic-type qualifications – although much work remains to be done here and those responsible for strategic policy tasks often find that appropriate training support is not readily available. Through dedicated journals, newsletters, reference libraries, web portals and training material, much research and experience are documented and made available. However, the less formal area of on-the-job training and knowledge exchange between practitioners based on individual experience is relatively poorly served. In the past, this was the primary source of knowledge for practical emergency management and arguably worked as long as there was low staff turnover and a range of mechanisms for such exchanges. This area of knowledge management remains critical to sound practice, but is often overlooked or ignored. Its major limitations are in the strategic area and, as mentioned above, with complex unbounded problems.

There are many international efforts at education and training for disaster reduction and risk management, driven by national aid agencies and NGOs such as Oxfam and Caritas, as well as numerous smaller faith-based and secular groups. Some fire and emergency management agencies link directly with their equivalents in poorer countries to provide training and equipment (e.g. Australian fire agencies have each paired with a fire agency in a south-west Pacific island country).

In addition, multilateral organizations are providing increasing leadership. Following on from the 1990s International Decade for Natural Disaster Reduction, the UN established the International Strategy for Disaster Reduction (ISDR) within the UN's Department of Humanitarian Affairs. The ISDR has produced the *Hyogo Framework* to set priorities and guide its work, and since late 2006 has been working with the World Bank's Global Facility for Disaster Reduction and Recovery. The fundamental aim of these multilateral agencies is to enhance capacity. Identifying risks though research and creating understanding and awareness through education are among the five priorities of the *Hyogo Framework* (UN–ISDR, 2004). Many of these international groups are dedicated to basic human development and see emergency management in that context, with an emphasis on building resilience.

Prospects for learning

Emergency managers and their organizations may be very effective learners (as those at risk can be); but application of the knowledge is largely contingent on the institutional context within which these entities operate. In this book, our concern is with this context, which is expanded on in Chapter 8. Institutions may be formal or informal, they may facilitate learning and improvement, or they may block learning. Institutional settings open to learning may be challenging to many who actively resist new knowledge – such knowledge can be threatening, suggesting change to those who do not want change since it may alter their status or business prospects, or require additional effort. Disciplinary views have long been seen as rejecting knowledge from other areas, with the result that solutions are similarly restricted. In the UK, engineers and finance department officials have, for decades, ensured that only a limited range of approaches to flood risk management (major engineering works) receive funding. This was not deliberate, but simply an outcome of an institutionalized strict cost-benefit analysis requirement for flood-related projects, which led to the production of detailed manuals by both the UK's Flood Hazard Research Centre and the Ministry of Agriculture, Fisheries and Food (MAFF), now known as the Department for Environment, Food and Rural Affairs (DEFRA).

Institutions are also crucial to applying knowledge: a population at risk and organizations that do not believe in their ability to influence outcomes are unlikely to see the point of learning and change. These are some of the institutional barriers that have to be overcome if a culture of learning is to be established. A culture of learning is of limited value itself in the absence of a culture of 'continuous improvement', which allows the learning to become action. Recalling the case studies in Chapter 1, Hurricane Katrina (see Box 1.1) illustrates some of the issues here, where the symbols of learning were present but the results very limited. The London smog showed learning, but over a massive span of time (see Box 1.9), whereas evacuation policy in Australian bushfires saw learning compressed into a shorter, although still arguably lengthy, period of time (see Box 1.4). Excepting the most extreme and unpredictable events, there are insights and lessons available to inform preparation and the reduction of vulnerability. The choice of whether policy learning occurs is largely a human one, not a random opportunity.

Notes

1 This discussion draws on elements of the extensive public policy literature on policy learning: see, for example, Bennett and Howlett (1992), May (1992), Lee (1993), Sabatier and Jenkins-Smith (1993) and Rose (2005).

2 It is accepted that 'commercial in confidence' or privacy considerations may be appropriate in some circumstances and that accessibility of information may therefore be limited. However, it should be the case that this is a necessary exception, rather than an immediate fall-back position or defensive strategy, in the interests of engagement by community and of accountability and efficiency in agency performance. The onus of proof should be on those wishing to maintain limited access to data, rather than those with a valid use in mind who wish to access the data.

8

Institutional Settings for Emergencies and Disasters: Form, Function and Coordination

Human societies achieve common goals and reconcile differences through the institutions that they create or inherit, whether those institutions are effective or not, constructive or destructive, democratic or autocratic, well informed or ignorant, formal or informal. Emergency managers and organizations charged with preparing for and managing disasters largely do an admirable and crucially important job. However, this task can only be performed as well as the institutional system within which these people and organizations are embedded, enabled and constrained allows it to be. We argue that insufficient attention has been paid to higher-order policy and institutional settings for emergencies and disasters, and note how the issue of institutions has emerged consistently throughout previous chapters.

This penultimate chapter gathers together issues and arguments about institutional settings for emergencies and disasters. It focuses mainly on the higher levels of those components of the governing state summarized in Table 2.1 in Chapter 2, but with reference to how these influence the crucial operational components and outcomes – institutions are a means to those ends. The chapter first revisits the concept of institution before summarily reviewing the common institutional settings in the field and some key problems and challenges experienced with those settings. Principles are then developed to inform the process of matching institutions with their purpose. A brief discussion of the role of law – an overlooked but critical factor in disasters policy – follows before concluding with an emphasis on the idea of coordination within the institutional system.

Institutions: The key to common endeavours

There is very little covered in this book thus far that can be achieved in the absence of appropriate institutional settings or understood without close analysis of that setting. Humans only achieve common goals, or satisfactorily reconcile differences, through institutions. To recall the definitions from Chapter 2:

- *Institutions* are persistent, predictable arrangements, laws, processes or customs serving to structure transactions and relationships in a society. These transactions include political, social, cultural, economic, personal, legal and administrative matters. Institutions may be informal or formal, legal or customary, and in terms of function may be economic, cultural or informational, highly visible and regulatory, or, alternatively, difficult to discern and relying on tacit understanding and adherence. Institutions allow organized, collective efforts around common concerns, and reduce the need for constant negotiation of expectations and behavioural contracts. Although persistent, institutions constantly evolve and adapt.

• The concept of an *institutional system* conveys the reality that concentrating on single institutions will often limit understanding. Institutions operate within complex interactive systems comprising multiple institutions, organizations and actors. Describing, analysing or prescribing policy change must take this interdependency into account.

Often, there is the apparent and recognized institutional system, but also a shadow system or less apparent institutions that need to be understood in order to expose how things really work. These multiple levels bedevil much risk management as the formal or official system may give a misleading picture of what the risk is. Often, emergency and risk management succeeds despite its institutional setting, where those responsible use their personal networks and informal or unofficial strategies to get the job done. Strategic planning and policy typically ignore this reality, but can acknowledge and incorporate such network capacities and become more flexible and robust as a result.

In emergency management theory and practice, most attention is paid to the role and functioning of *organizations*, the more tangible manifestations of underlying institutions. Similarly, attention is paid to management prescriptions and regulations, rather than to strategic policy directions. Differentiating between these is, at times, difficult: for example, management activities are influenced by policy and vice versa. An organization or even individual may be sufficiently long lived, recognized and influential to be regarded as an institution – consider the seven-term mayor or the long-standing local volunteer fire brigade. The colloquial understanding of 'institution', implying consistency and visibility of a presence and influence, is not that different from the theoretical understanding mirrored in the first sentence of the definition above.

The second definition – institutional system – defines a core theme of this chapter and of the challenge of coping with disasters. The precise form and quality of any one institutional component responsible for an aspect of disaster policy and response is only as important as the form and quality of the interactions with other components. It is precisely this institutional interdependency and coordination, and the strategic policy processes and settings that shape them (and, therefore, the capacity to persist, learn and improve) that are the big challenge. The prompt arrival of military services for evacuation in a disaster is crucial, but is determined not only by the preparedness and professionalism of the military units, but by the clear definition of decision-making in government, the quality of transport infrastructure and other factors. However, a number of institutions are needed for effective emergency management: those dedicated to community safety and resilience are often poorly resourced compared with response, perhaps not surprisingly given the political imperative of sound response.

A fine-resolution local government planning scheme that accounts for community resilience and vulnerability to disasters and that may minimize exposure and maintain livelihoods is a good thing, but is not effective if under constant legal challenge, unimplemented due to lack of resources or unenforceable due to weak regulatory capacities and illegal land use. A well-designed long-term aid programme to diversify livelihoods and enhance resilience will not achieve its desired outcomes in the face of weak or corrupt local institutions (or local institutions with different priorities), and serviceable institutions in a very poor community can do little without positive contributions from outside. In terms of emergency management, this argues for a uniform approach across jurisdictions rather than an approach entirely dependent on local resources and capacities. For example, such communities may not have the resources for basic fire protection, with the result that each fire leaves the community even poorer (Lynn, 2003).

As whole-of-society and whole-of-government problems, emergencies and disasters require connected institutional elements to be linked to policy processes. Consider some of the case studies from Chapter 1 (see Boxes 1.1 to 1.9).

Dedicated institutions are inadequate: Hurricane Katrina in New Orleans

The emergency management system had rehearsed the event well, but somehow it just did not connect with local realities and vulnerabilities; neither was there adequate information flow for decision-making in the context of the existing system. In practice, there was very limited cooperation between agencies, the three levels of government and major NGO relief groups. Informal connections – the shadow system – did not fill the gap. Some commentators have observed that there was a serious inability to adapt to exceptionally complex circumstances. There is also the issue of what the aim of much of the emergency management system was directed towards – security or relief – and the extent to which this is embedded in the American approach. The US Coast Guard operated effectively in this environment and may provide a useful guide.

Institution of economic recovery leaves many out: The South Asian tsunami

In southern Thailand, the central government's strategic recovery plan paid special attention to local businesses and to the flows of money that make the local economy vibrant. It did this rather than emphasize highly visible actions, such as the reconstruction of buildings. In doing so, however, it was trapped within the normal institution of economic thinking and ignored the informal or undocumented economy. The informal economy provides employment for some one third to half of the people of southern Thailand, and is how the economy really works for many people. Their livelihood recovery hinges on it.

Changing a fundamental institution: Wildfire safety in Australia

The fact that responsibility for many risks is shared is almost orthodoxy in policy documents; however, certain key aspects of emergency management institutions suggest that it may be otherwise. Australian fire authorities have worked to make shared responsibility real through the 'Stay or Go' approach (or, more fully, 'prepare, stay and defend, or leave early'), in which able-bodied residents are encouraged to consider staying with their homes as a wildfire front passes. The approach is based on research showing that most fatalities were due to people being caught in the fire when evacuating late. This is contradictory to the traditional ethos of the emergency service, which is immediate evacuation. It has taken several decades; but the development of a national, more evidence-based, approach to fire management and community safety has led to all fire agencies endorsing 'prepare, stay and defend, or leave early'. The current institutional challenge concerns bringing other agencies on board and achieving full implementation.

Incorporating multiple objectives: Flood management in The Netherlands

In The Netherlands, societal institutions dedicated – as the centuries-old dominant national priority – to keeping water out have evolved to accommodate the idea that there could be 'space for rivers' and even the sea, on occasions. This reflects changing attitudes and a strong belief reflected in politics that environmental imperatives should be accommodated along with safety. There are substantial financial savings to be derived from this approach as well. It may also be partly a result of the time that has elapsed since the last serious sea flooding during the early 1950s, although the standards of protection are in legislation.

Institutions and emergencies: Status and issues

In these examples, we see the necessary but often missing or imperfect connections between different elements of the institutional system. Some of these elements are well recognized as crucial to the business of emergency response; others are usually perceived as less relevant, but indirectly very influential. The following section identifies the core agencies and players – the 'usual suspects' of emergency management – and then describes the institutional landscape more widely in order to identify a larger range of elements.

These well-recognized elements of the institutional setting of emergency and disaster policy and management are, however, only part of the *institutional system* that enables or constrains how well societies can understand, prepare for and handle disruption and surprise. Table 8.1 significantly extends the 'components of the governing state' presented in Table 2.1 and portrays the key components of the institutional system within which disasters are understood, debated and addressed. Note that while the components are defined separately, all are intricately interdependent – a core issue discussed further below.

Table 8.1 *Components of the institutional system (expanding upon Table 2.1), with typical roles regarding emergencies and disasters*

Component	Role	Examples in emergencies and disasters (direct and indirect relevance to emergencies)
Constitution, political system	Definition of rules and boundaries of responsibilities within the institutional system	Division of responsibilities between national and sub-national governments; definition of recourse to judiciary
Executive and legislature	Debate of social goals, law-making, policy development and institutional change	President and/or prime minister, cabinet, outer ministry, political staff and advisers, formulating disasters policy
Public service departments	Inform and implement government policy Line departments with particular roles; central agencies with whole-of-government roles	Various portfolios directly or indirectly relevant to disasters: health, infrastructure, police, justice, defence, science, environment, transport, regional development and biosafety
Statutory authorities and other semi-autonomous public agencies	Government functions deemed ongoing in nature, requiring independence, consistency over time and distance from political control	Emergency services authorities, land management (e.g. forests) authorities, the military, auditors general and the ambulance service
Judicial bodies	Interpretation and application of laws Recommend changes in the law and procedures	Coroner courts, commissions of inquiry, administrative courts, etc.; function of review and scrutiny post-disaster
Enforcement and regulatory agencies	Monitoring and enforcement of laws and regulations (sometimes one function of a department or statutory authority)	Police, health and building inspectors, maritime safety inspectors, environmental protection agencies
(In federal systems, state or provincial governments)	*(Similar, in various relationships to national governments)*	*(Similar, with extensive variation according to constitutional and political distribution of powers)*

Table 8.1 *Continued*

Component	Role	Examples in emergencies and disasters (direct and indirect relevance to emergencies)
Local government	Functions vary widely: service delivery, planning and development, library and information services, infrastructure provision, etc.	Building code application; land-use planning; management of reserves, roads, water and waste management, foreshores, etc.; information provision and community education
Intergovernmental bodies (within one country)	Coordination of roles and responsibilities across governments (vertical or horizontal); cross-jurisdictional policy and management functions	National fire councils, emergency services agencies, coordinated public health response agreements, river basin management bodies
International organizations, institutions and agreements	Coordination of activities, standard-setting, policy and management of issues beyond individual jurisdictional competence	Various United Nations bodies, international financial institutions, international treaties, development aid agencies, international scientific bodies and disaster response agreements between countries (all may be global, regional or bilateral)
Public trading corporations	Government-owned or government-controlled trading corporations, also known as government business enterprises (GBEs)	Water authorities, corporate resource management agencies (e.g. forest agencies, land commissions), some banks, telecommunications bodies and postal services
Private firms	Profit-oriented entities, small or large, cooperative or resistant to policy and regulatory directions, often required to implement these directions	Land development interests, rural producers, builders, architects, private infrastructure providers, consultants, engineering firms, petro-chemical firms and fire equipment manufacturers

Table 8.1 *Continued*

Component	Role	Examples in emergencies and disasters (direct and indirect relevance to emergencies)
Industry associations	Organizations representing professions, sectors, etc. with communication, self-regulatory and advocacy functions	Farmers' organizations, and forest industry, oil transport, etc. associations involved in policy debate, preparedness and response regarding disasters; lobby for particular practices
Semi-state institutions	Various groupings, often supported or regulated by government, involved in policy debates and service delivery	Hospitals, disaster relief charitable organizations, relevant university research centres, religious institutions, labour organizations, NGO advocacy groups
Media (public or private)	Dissemination of information and/or opinion in community, political advocacy, etc.; local, regional, national and international	Communication of disaster-related information, mediators and initiators of policy debates, reportage of agency performance, advocates of policy change
Epistemic communities (groups defined by expertise)	Knowledge- or expertise-based groups and networks providing information, setting research and policy agendas and advocating policy positions	Infrastructure engineers, wildlife ecologists, hydrologists, epidemiologists, development studies, economic analysts, risk assessment experts
Informal and community-based institutions and organizations	Local-scale organizations, networks and rules/norms, some formal and recognizable, some intangible (may be linked to formal agencies of the state)	Local socially enforced customs, neighbourhood fire-watch groups, kinship networks, co-operatives, volunteer fire or emergency service brigades
Other NGOs (non-governmental organizations or non-profits) Levels from international to local/community	Range from advocacy for individuals to major political change, fundraising and transfer, and practical action	Transfer expertise and funds to poorer areas to build resilience and disaster zones to help recovery

Source: Expanded from Davis et al (1993)

In keeping with the definition in Chapter 2 of an institutional system, only partially useful consideration can be given to any one of these levels in isolation: rarely will one act or fulfil its function without connection to others. Local governments play important roles in emergency management in many jurisdictions, but in a manner enabled or constrained by the statutory and fiscal settings created by a state or provincial government, and in close cooperation with a higher-level emergency bureau and with local informal community groups. A cabinet-level policy decision is subject to the overview of judicial deliberation, if challenged, and will be formulated and especially implemented in concert with line departments. Statutory authorities are subject to some government oversight and by the decisions of central agencies, such as a prime minister's department or treasury. Virtually all activities by any actors are influenced by the interest and style of coverage of media organizations, whether well communicated or well received by the broader community.

Major issues experienced with current institutional settings include lack of coordination between agencies; ownership of policy by a few with subsequent domination of narrow perspectives; poor information generation and exchange; political interference and the issue of what policy objectives really are; ability to cope with complexity and high levels of uncertainty; lack of flexibility; over-reliance on poorly supported volunteerism; and issues of human resources.

Lack of coordination between agencies is one perennial finding of post-disaster inquiries – the institutional setting more often than not discourages information-sharing, cooperation and all that follows on from this. These issues are by no means limited to relations between agencies; they occur within agencies, as well, often because those with responsibility for working across the parts of agencies, as well as between agencies, have very low status and can be seen as irritants – the institutional arrangements as played out, as opposed to what is on paper, do not support them. This can be reflected in the often weak support for, and ownership of, policy as it is developed in isolation from those who would ideally own and implement it.

Meeting the changing expectations of the communities being served, and working with those communities in sharing responsibility for the risk, is another central problem for existing institutional structures that evolved during a period when such wider participation was not as common. Accepting and dealing with high levels of complexity and uncertainty are major challenges and ones for which obvious solutions do not exist. Effort directed towards creating an ability to work with limited information, such as frequently occurs during a crisis, should help. Earlier, we argued that attention to flexibility and adaptability is of value – but the emphasis in many emergency institutions remains on command and control, with its tendency to rigidity. No matter how well organized such tightly controlled processes are, and whatever the views of emergency planners and managers, flexibility is needed, at minimum, because operation objectives are often compromised by changing political imperatives.

There is also a strong push from some quarters for change – but change concerning greatly expanded use of modern technology and public education, rather than more fundamental institutional changes. Of course, technology and education have important roles to play, but will not achieve their promise if unsupported by, and embedded in, the institutional system as core parts of an integrated strategic approach. These quite well-known problems with existing arrangements can be viewed from the perspective of choices of policy styles and institutional strategy – continua with contrasting extremes that will be variously championed or pilloried by different actors. There is the continuum between the institutional choices of placing something in the more direct political control of a line department, with the risk of reaction to short-term imperatives only, versus the independence and greater longevity of a potentially unresponsive statutory authority. Similarly, there is a continuum between strong mechanisms for (vertical and/or horizontal) whole-of-government coordination, with a risk of dissipating efforts through the coordination processes, versus the possibly clearer purpose and development of control and capacity in specific agencies, but with less coordination. The benefits of paramilitary discipline and clarity can be considered versus the democratic benefits and operational uncertainties of civic engagement, or the human capacity issue through cheaper volunteerism versus more costly career personnel. The need for persistence of efforts and expertise across events, however organizationally achieved, may appear in contrast to the need for flexibility and back-up capacity attained through different organizational structures. Information requirements can be handled through centralized information systems (which are reliable but prone to a lack of context specificity and are vulnerable to the whims of budget cycles) or through greater emphasis on networks and local knowledge, perhaps more resilient but certainly more complex to construct and maintain. If the argument for institutional (separate from operational) redundancy and fail safes is accepted, this stands in contrast to imperatives of efficiency.

This begs the question of the 'mainstreaming' of disaster policy to embed disasters across policy sectors as a core consideration, and to guard against the tendency to neglect disaster policy when considerable time has elapsed since the last event. The use of independent statutory emergency agencies has great merits, but can remove issues from the mainstream of policy and politics. On the other hand, too much responsibility placed within traditional government departments and, especially, in powerful central agencies risks politicization and rapid, poorly conceived shifts of agenda. A balance and combination of both, along with other strategies, is advisable, with multiple nodes of responsibility, capacity and information. The redundancy and spare capacity that high stakes and great uncertainty invite is not just operational, but also institutional.

In a similar vein, few institutional choices are binary. Even the end points of these various continua of institutional and policy style – the extremes – have their place at particular junctures and times. Reacting purposefully in the face of on oncoming disaster event, or during one, requires very different policy style and institutional forms than those suitable for discussing community resilience strategies at the local level. Where massive variability in events, socio-economic context, spatial scale, response capacity, community resilience and political system is the norm, and where multiple interests, roles, actors and responsibilities are engaged – as in emergency management – a variety of institutional structures and processes is clearly needed. Multiple management arrangements, policy processes, organizations and institutions will be engaged – whether effectively or not – in understanding, preparing for, responding to and recovering from disasters. The challenge is less which institutional strategy, but which ones, in what combination, for what purposes in particular environmental and socio-economic contexts.

Institutions as a means to an end

Institutions are a way of achieving something: they are a means to an end, whatever that end or goal is – economic growth, human health, national security, community resilience, sensibly laid-out towns, or protecting lives and livelihoods from disasters. Institutions are often overlooked, but they are not ends in themselves. Arguing for one or another institutional or organizational form without reference to its purpose or it merits relative to other forms treats institutions as ends rather than means.

This applies not only to proposed institutional and organizational settings, but to existing settings when they are being questioned or reviewed. Those within an institutional system, particularly in long-standing organizations, may focus on the survival of the organization as an end in itself, forgetting the role that society expects of it and expects to be paramount, or assuming that the organization is the only way of performing that role. To be defensive when doubt is cast on us is a natural human reaction, individually and collectively, and critical constructive reflection is a hard thing to manage. Methods are required to clarify the divide between the who (did it), the what and the why (it happened), utilizing different approaches to attribute blame and the more creative and constructive exercise of driving improvement.

An overarching principle in considering better institutional settings for emergencies and disasters is to *consider institutional function before form*. While an enduring and well-recognized institution or powerful organization should not be torn down or radically revised unthinkingly (it is there and has survived for a reason), nor should it be accepted uncritically, without reference to performance in acquitting the role that society expects of it. The multiple values and roles of the many actors and organizations with a part to play in disaster policy tell us that simple function–form choices are few: multiple activities and responsibilities are scattered across multiple interacting components of a complex institutional system. The question reappears, already raised above, concerning the advantages and disadvantages of a line department over the independence of a statutory authority. Public agencies have many functions, and the answer to this question will vary according to which function is under consideration. This is a standard question in public administration; but in the emergency management field, it is complicated greatly by those familiar attributes of pervasive uncertainty, cross-sectoral connectivity, awkward scales of time and space, and obscure rights and responsibilities. Does it, for example, make sense for a major evacuation in the face of an immediate threat to require high-level government approval? For what functions is local volunteerism the most appropriate response as opposed to organizations with career professionals, in what combination and within what broader organizational and institutional setting?

The following section steps back from the operational and structural questions to explore generic principles for informing the analysis and design of institutions for emergencies and disasters, drawing on ideas from the institutional literature and the related domain of sustainability in a manner consistent with the particular challenges presented by emergency management.

Purpose, form and principles

The characteristics of an institutional setting should reflect the purpose, and as purposes vary greatly, a range of design principles should be considered. In a general discussion such as this book, it is not possible to specify the features of specific institutional settings. However, the field of institutional theory and design offers general principles that apply to human institutions broadly, and which serve as a starting point for considering institutional design for emergency management. Goodin (1996) offers the following 'design principles' that reflect the attributes of institutions that are successful in that they persist over time and fulfil their mandate (whether one agrees with that mandate or not):

- *adaptability* (being capable of change in evolving situations);
- *robustness* so as not to be liable to change too swiftly or unthinkingly;
- *recognition of, and sensitivity to*, complexity in motivations of individuals and groups, ensuring congruence with expectations of different groups interacting with the institution;
- *being publicly defensible*, ensuring political and social support;
- *variability* (being able to experiment with different structures in different places).

These are general but important features of institutions of any kind, and are useful reference points for assessing an existing institution or proposing institutional reform.

It can be too easy to think of institutions in only structural terms, forgetting that they are parts of society, conceived of and run by human beings. Dryzek (1996) differentiates between institutional 'hardware' and 'software'. The former is the actual form and structure of the institution, the latter the knowledge, practices, cultural norms, etc. that make it work. This differentiation is critically important in emergencies and disasters since it is often informal or personal knowledge and networks that enable successful preparedness and response.

Another set of features of 'adaptive' institutions can be gleaned from resource and environmental management – a similar policy sector to emergency management. The following requirements, adapted from Chapter 3, both extend and emphasize some of Goodin's general principles (Dovers, 2005):

- *persistence*, allowing sufficient time for policy and institutional 'experiments' to be run and lessons accrued: too rapid or constant institutional and organizational change generally results in loss of continuity, institutional memory and the ability to learn and evolve;
- *purposefulness*, or a common sense of purpose and mission, through a widely recognized mandate and a set of core policy goals and principles;
- *information richness and sensitivity*, especially maintained over time: this refers not only to information gathering, but to the wide distribution, broad ownership and appropriate use of information;
- *inclusiveness*, or accessibility to relevant stakeholders, achieved through clearly

understood and sustained public participation in both higher-level policy and operational management;
- *flexibility* to balance persistence and purposefulness, and to ensure that they do not develop into rigidity, but allow adaptation and learning.

These attributes may seem obvious; but it is not apparent that they are always considered or achieved in the assessment or design of institutional settings. Importantly, they are not strict 'rules' and need to be balanced against each other – for example, persistence versus flexibility. In addition, their interpretation and application will vary greatly across different contexts, involving a level of detail not possible here.

Another interesting principle is the suitability of 'goodness of fit' in institutional design: a feature of influential long-lived institutions is that they fit in their operating environment (Goodin, 1996). This is an obvious element of accepted functioning institutions. Yet, in the case of disasters, the 'operating environment' during and after events will, by definition, be *abnormal* and in complex events, at least, will change rapidly – thus, an institutional setting for disasters will likely be at odds with 'normal' expectations of institutions, as well as the criteria against which public institutions are usually judged. While an institution may eventually acquit its disaster-related functions splendidly in the abnormal operating environment of an event, it may also be assessed and judged, even attacked, under normal conditions – a time when it may appear strange and even at odds with economic development or government ideology, for example, by attempting to restrict floodplain development or to provide information on industrial hazards. This means that the differences between a disaster-competent institution and other institutions must be identified and justified.

One way of exploring this tension is to consider the stability or changeability of an institution through a coarse-scale categorization of different forms of *institutional resilience*, which is the way in which it responds to external change and stimuli (Handmer and Dovers, 1996):

- *Type 1 resilience: Resistance and maintenance*. This strategy is characterized positively by purpose and stability, optimization of resource use and a low risk of ill-considered change. Negatively, it is characterized by denial of, or resistance to, change, appeals to ignorance, awaiting crisis before reforming operating assumptions and practices, and unlikely to be effective in prevention and preparedness activities or at achieving cross-government or multiple-sector commitment to emergency management. Nevertheless, it is probably effective for routine events.
- *Type 2 resilience: Change at the margins*. This resilience is positively characterized by the admission of a need for change, well-considered reactions to outside pressures and new situations, and manageable incremental responses. It is negatively characterized by the inability to cope with major shifts in the operating environment or by new knowledge, addressing symptoms rather than causes; by the lack of a long-term strategy; and by the danger of masking the continuation of a problem through the veneer of change. This is a common approach that

provides a sense of stability, while paying some attention to needed change, and may often be the best that can be achieved.
- *Type 3 resilience: Openness and adaptability.* This strategy is positively characterized by recognition of uncertainty and imperatives for change (including addressing underlying causes) and by preparedness to adapt quickly. It is negatively characterized by inefficiency and possible maladaptation through poorly considered change. This is a very important attribute when faced with a complex unbounded problem and limited resources. In prevention and preparedness, it may be very useful in gaining support and working across different sectors.

All three forms of resilience are appropriate in different circumstances: the problem faced, the state of knowledge and the implications of not taking action. Different institutions and individuals tend to favour one form and to criticize the adequacy of other strategies. The nature of emergencies and disasters, especially pervasive uncertainty, suggests that a disaster-competent institution must have the capacity to be able to entertain – often in haste – and adopt a suitable strategy according to the situation confronting it. In a threatening and fluid operating environment, 'resistance and maintenance' would generally be regarded as a dangerous propensity; however, in routine emergencies, it may be optimal. Likewise, 'change at the margin' may be successful in the face of non-routine or meso events, but serve to develop an assumed level of safety – designed-in disasters. 'Openness and adaptability' may seem the obvious strategy in disaster situations, but does carry the risk of maladaptation.

What emerges here is that for emergency management institutions, a single institution or set of institutions should assess what resilience strategies are best suited to *specific aspects* of their structure and function, rather than favouring one strategy as a general rule.

Emergency management institutions in practice

Mechanisms to achieve or improve institutional function include attempts at changing structure through unifying the major emergency management type agencies, and the use of coordinating authorities superimposed on the existing institutional structure. Distinct agencies may, nevertheless, function cooperatively in some areas through networks of personal contacts or shared personnel. In many countries, attempts are being made to reduce the importance of such networks through training, operating procedures and technology. However, personal networks help to provide the flexibility and adaptability needed to make emergency management work, especially for problems outside the 'routine'. The reality in most of the world is that informal networks will remain important, in part, because the institutions are not conducive to the changes needed to find substitutes. The informal provides the flexibility denied by the obvious structures.

Often, institutional failures, and opportunities for reform, exist at the boundaries of spatial and administrative scale. Most pronounced in federal systems, this is frequently apparent between the formal levels of government: local, provincial and national. However, issues of scale can arise within a level of government, such as when different policy sectors (health, communications, defence, etc.) are organized within different regional boundaries. In civil society, issues of uncoordinated or well-coordinated scale may arise between international, national and local NGOs, and in the commercial world between international headquarters and local offices and franchises.

Disasters rarely respect administrative boundaries, and so the boundaries of government and administration may be barriers to understanding disasters and to effective preparation and response. The spatial boundaries of emergency management policy may be, for most other policy concerns, strange and illogical – vegetation type for wildfires, river corridors for flooding, demographic groups for epidemics – and difficult to support or reconcile administratively. Yet, should administrative boundaries be considered sacrosanct, then vulnerability to events will likely increase.

Whatever the formal structure, emergency management is expected to encompass an increasing variety of agencies, sectors and interests: this is much more than 'whole of government' – it approaches 'whole of society'. Failure to engage with the wider range of groups is likely to see formal emergency management organizations reduced to playing a part role, with essential work left undone.

Learning, law and liability

Institutions create powerful incentives and disincentives for learning and behaviour, although the incentives may not be well aligned with emergency management. Two of the overarching institutional mechanisms in most societies are economics and the law: the actions of most stakeholders in most situations need to be legally and economically defensible.

Law gains power as an instrument of learning and change through its ability to enforce sanctions against individuals and organizations – something most of us learn to avoid. Such sanctions may be of a criminal nature, with the state bringing court action; those who suffer loss as a result of actions may also go to court, seeking compensation through civil procedures. Administrative law is also important in relation to breaches of regulations, such as safety, planning and health. The threat of court sanctions is a powerful persuader, but may make emergency management cautious, slow to issue warnings and reluctant to provide critical advice. Courts of both common law and civil code jurisdictions view rescue and emergency management as desirable and generally support the activities of those involved in response. However, the law as imagined may be as influential as law actioned in the courts. The result is that, in many jurisdictions, an unfortunate and incorrect view is that emergency workers (whether spontaneous, trained volunteers or career professionals) may be found legally liable by those whom they rescue, making many people needlessly cautious about assisting others in an emergency. Occasionally, law can force revolutionary change, at least on paper; but practice can resist and subvert the legal intent.

Perhaps paradoxically, emergency management may find that the law is of limited help when arguing for a precautionary approach to development, or when attempting to enhance community resilience. In these more strategic circumstances, law and economic imperatives often coalesce to sideline emergency management concerns. Economic or 'market' factors, such as taxation, fees and charges, and the price of land and insurance, may act to encourage or discourage appropriate action by commercial entities, as well as individuals. An obvious example concerns incentives to develop hazardous land. Of course, in many cases, people have little option but to occupy such locations faced with the need to gain livelihoods and housing, regardless of the legalities. The informal or shanty towns of many cities testify to this. Laws might mandate the provision of improved housing in low hazard areas; but the people involved often have to live adjacent to their livelihoods. Resolving the issue of which emphasis makes the greater contribution to resilience is difficult. For examples where law has acted in these circumstances, see Handmer and Monson (2004). Less obvious is the full commercialization of essential services, such as electricity or gas, where it becomes more profitable for the company to sell the product to another jurisdiction during a period of high demand, leaving an area without reliable supply. Law from areas apparently far from the immediate concerns of emergency management may nevertheless be very important.

Changes to both the legal and economic frameworks can arise from inquiries conducted after a disaster. Typically, post-disaster inquiries are quasi-legal in form and too often focus on the attribution of blame and protection of elected officials. As a result, important recommendations are easily overlooked or, if accepted, starved through lack of resourcing. This is not always the case, and many inquiries are conducted in the spirit of learning and improvement.

The final, and often overlooked, role of law is the codification of social values and goals as objectives and responsibilities in statute law. Agency staff will address those functions assigned to them in enabling legislation before any additional and non-compulsory coordination functions; therefore, if inter-agency coordination is agreed as required, then enabling legislation should recognize and mandate such work. The law plays a fundamental role in structuring the institutional system and should be a key player in discussions of institutional change.

Conclusion

There are as many institutional options for dealing with disasters as there are policy instruments (see Chapter 6), and none are inherently superior or generically applicable. Nevertheless, the choice matters: the needs of a specific context can define more precisely the institutional settings most likely to reduce vulnerability and to react effectively to the unexpected or feared. As disasters are framed as more and more a whole-of-society issue, the range of actual institutions and options expands. In reality, there will always be a number of distinct formal and informal emergency management institutions in any given place and time. Most will overlap to some degree; but some, such as those in other countries, may not. Some will be connected and cooperate; others may not. In the face of varied and uncertain events, the institutional framework needs to be open and adaptable in the mode and scale of its operation, but sufficiently predictable to be relied on. It needs to be able to adapt to a very wide range of priorities and circumstances: prevention of routine emergencies demands different skills and strategies in response and recovery than a large-scale complex event with explicit international dimensions.

A major challenge in institutional design is being able to link with and coordinate diverse groups, as needed, for different problems and circumstances, including international linkages, those in the commercial world and a range of NGOs. Perhaps more difficult is the ability to work with all groups in society, including those normally invisible, such as undocumented workers, institutionalized populations and the semi-literate.

The greatest task in this sense is not the specific design of singular institutional mechanisms, even if the poor design and subsequent failure of one such mechanism may have tragic consequences. It is the recognition of the more complex institutional system and the coordination and optimal function of that system.

Part III

Constructing the Future

9

Future Prospects

This concluding chapter focuses on apparent and important inadequacies in contemporary emergency management, and considers some trends that are worrying in terms of future disasters, revisiting Chapter 1 in the process. The potential consequences of increasing disaster risk and inadequate capacities are briefly examined. Trends in policy thinking are also discussed. The final section brings these together, with suggestions of where policy may provide the most help to emergency management in meeting likely challenges.

How disastrous a future?

For those concerned about climatic hazards, the news is not good. *Climate Change 2007*, the latest Intergovernmental Panel on Climate Change (IPCC) report has just been released, following close on the heels of the UK's Stern Report on the economic impacts of climate change. Both paint a grim picture:

> Warming of the global climate is unequivocal ... numerous long-term changes in climate have been observed. These include ... aspects of extreme weather, including droughts, heavy precipitation, heat waves and the intensity of tropical cyclones... These are very likely to become more frequent. (IPCC 2007)

The Economics of Climate Change: The Stern Review (Stern et al, 2006) emphasizes that the world has to act now or 'face devastating economic consequences'. On 17 April 2007, the UK put climate change on the agenda of the United Nations Security Council, arguing that it threatened global security. This was not supported by all Security Council members, but follows a number of reports carrying similar warnings – for example, a report by the US Center for Naval Analysis (2007) and a London conference quoted from the BBC:

> Global warming could exacerbate the world's rich–poor divide and help to radicalize populations and fan terrorism in the countries worst affected, security and climate experts said on Wednesday. 'We have to reckon with the human

propensity for violence', Sir Crispin Tickell, Britain's former ambassador to the United Nations, told a London Conference on Climate Change: The Global Security Impact. (RUSI, 2007)

These scientific reports and comments, and many like them, are strongest on the changes reflected in technical climatic and weather measurements, and the reasons for these. However, for many people, especially those living in the northern arctic, sub-arctic and temperate regions, the changes to their environments have been dramatic (CIEL, 2007), threatening livelihoods and, in some cases, people's existence. The potential impacts on the hundreds of millions living at or near sea level have been the main focus of mainstream climate change scenarios. Added to the threat of sea-level rise is the possibility of more cyclones (hurricanes/typhoons) and floods, and, in other areas, extended droughts and permanent water deficits. The impacts on agriculture of higher temperatures and more frequent extremes, including large wildfires, may undermine food production and threaten to shift some areas to a state of permanent crisis. Storm intensity is likely to increase in many areas.

Changes or variability in the climate are only part of the picture, however. Widespread environmental and water contamination is likely in the future, related to disruption through weather events, but also simply from expanding population and industrialization, putting more people closer to more hazardous industries and contaminants.

As set out in Chapter 1, it is trends in the exposure and vulnerability of people that are (or should be) firmly within the ambit of emergency management. If they are not, emergency management is likely to be constrained to responding to emergencies of escalating scale and complexity. Many of these trends were discussed in Chapter 1, some of which are listed below:

- *Population increase and, importantly, its distribution:* globally, this affects a dispro-portionate number of poor people, dependants (children and youth) and people living in hazardous locations with marginal livelihoods.
- *Urbanization* creates mass concentrations of humans and economic activity: the potential for most types of emergencies is increased, with greater impacts on more people; but simultaneously, the capacity to plan and deal with them may be increased.
- *Conflict,* whether over resources, ideologies, ethnic division or without clear rationale, destroys resilience by damaging livelihoods and food sources, forces mass displacement and redirects resources from productive use. Conflict creates crises while often undermining emergency management and other capacities to react.
- *The breakdown of governance and institutions* removes much capacity for organ-ized emergency management and undermines the resilience of economies and communities, whether through reduced capacity or rising corruption.
- *Uncertainty:* it appears that there is increasing uncertainty on all fronts, whether geophysical, economic, social values, political, legal or administrative.
- *Inequity and vulnerability:* in addition to the trends listed above, vulnerable groups are being created through employment conditions, access to healthcare and displacement for other forms of development.

We can reasonably ask how well emergency management does today, and whether it has the policy and institutional capacity to cope with these trends and forecasts. In summary – taking a broad definition of emergency management to include all involved, such as non-governmental groups – it does extraordinarily well in many parts of the world despite the fact that things occasionally go wrong even in well-resourced areas. Nevertheless, the picture is very patchy, with the emphasis generally on media-friendly, high-profile responses, and with limited attention given to other parts of the emergency management function: prevention, preparedness and long-term recovery. Addressing prevention, and improving resilience or reducing vulnerability, often requires fundamental change, challenges major power interests and may disrupt the status quo. Under these circumstances, it is therefore likely to be resisted. Failure to address this basic developmental challenge in many parts of the world will result in increasingly large losses of life, livelihoods, and economic assets and activity.

There is a plausible but worst-case scenario of far greater frequency and magnitude of emergencies and disasters, at all scales, in both rich and poor areas, and grossly insufficient capacities. However, scenarios that are less alarming, with negative impacts but of lesser magnitude, will, nonetheless, threaten emergency response capacity and still see increasing disruption and increasing pressures on society's ability to cope. So, all other things being equal, many areas will struggle to handle disasters in the future. The policy and institutional challenge may or may not be overwhelming; but it will certainly be far from trivial.

Viewed globally, key deficiencies with contemporary emergency management that limit abilities to deal with today's circumstances, and therefore even more so in the future, include:

- a preoccupation with response to particular events at the expense of other elements of emergency management;
- a lack of strategic policy development, leaving emergency managers and communities constrained within existing policy and institutional capacities;
- reorienting of emergency management to focus more on issues of national security, especially related to threats of terrorism, which may be at the expense of emergency management's capacity to deal with other, and generally larger, risks;
- privatization of emergency management functions with a consequent emphasis on profit rather than safety; this is seen in response and in some forms of prevention, rather than emphasizing all approaches, including the relatively low-cost measures taken by individuals;
- increasing issues of confidentiality that security and privatization bring, with consequent decline likely in cross-sector cooperation and accessibility of information and policy processes;
- difficulties in learning and capacity-building across events, and maintaining political mainstream profile and support;
- building resilience may be hindered by established interests; related to this is the question of the appropriate balance between anticipatory and resiliency approaches.

The question arises as to how stable these factors are. Could there be sudden change, with some becoming much more important or other factors appearing? The answer must be, yes, as evidenced by the counter-terrorism emphasis that appeared so immediately after the 11 September 2001 attacks in the US and, to a lesser extent, the sudden interest in tsunamis following the 26 December 2004 Asian event. Sudden climate impacts, disease outbreaks, civil or military conflict – any such disruptions, depending on where they impact – could reorient the policy discussion and direction. The reorientation could be positive, such as a focus on resilience in the wake of wider appreciation of the threats of climate change, or negative, such as a narrowing of the agenda to focus on security.

To further develop policy and institutional capacities in it own domain, emergency and disaster management – whether severely affected by these deficiencies or not – intersects with a broader policy environment driven by its own particular trends.

Policy styles vary from country to country and are not stable over time, so a detailed analysis is neither possible here, nor would it be likely to apply for long. Such volatility is normal in the political realm and is particularly pronounced in a policy domain such as disasters, where sudden events and reactions to them can shift agendas and priorities so quickly. Indeed, one challenge for the emergencies and disasters field is to maintain a close engagement within the policy community in order to be aware of shifts in policy style and therefore to be capable of responding to shifts, or even to influence policy shifts, rather than simply reacting after the fact. Such a 'mainstreaming' of disasters as a policy issue within the institutional system was discussed in Chapter 8. In monitoring shifts in the policy and institutional operating environment of emergency and disaster management, important trends in policy and institutional styles include the following balances between:

- public and private provision of policy advice, information, management services, etc. in relevant sectors affecting emergencies and disasters (the neo-liberal turn in public policy has profoundly influenced many sectors, and whether this trend will continue, stabilize or reverse will be an important determinant of policy approaches admitted and capacities that can be developed);
- specifically, the relative advocacy and acceptability of different policy instruments, and the choices between regulatory, self-regulatory, market-based, educative and community-based approaches (the balance between coercion, collaboration and sermonizing has shifted during recent decades and will doubtless continue to evolve);
- centralization and devolution of public policy and, thus, emergency management policy responsibilities and operational functions (this is also known as the *subsidiarity* debate in governance – including both the government and non-governmental sectors);
- types of policy formulation and the degree to which inclusive processes of policy *formulation* (as opposed to operational implementation) are encouraged or permitted, thus determining problem-framing and thereby the trajectory of instrument choice, implementation style, etc.;
- the responsibility and influence of international policy and institutions in the

disaster field versus that retained by national and sub-national levels;
- the relative weight given to other major social and policy issues, which may strengthen or diminish the priority and attention given to disasters (these issues include social equity, free trade, economic growth and efficiency, security, and environment and sustainability);
- in particular, the trend in economic and human development policy that ranges from the extremes of reliance on macro-economic (structural adjustment and institutional reform) to reliance on community-scale 'bottom-up' development and resilience.

Reflecting on this complex and unstable policy environment, and given that there is no reason to believe that event frequency and/or magnitude will decrease, but rather that it will noticeably increase, the future for disaster policy and its institutional setting lies somewhere between current inadequacies being somewhat exacerbated, and catastrophic breakdown of capacities. The next section identifies major policy and institutional challenges that can be expected if the future falls about midway between these extremes.

Key challenges

For all levels of emergencies, countries where governments seek legitimacy in the eyes of their citizens will generally be better served by emergency management. In large part, this is because such countries are likely to have institutions dedicated to the task of public safety that are reasonably effective, at least at the routine level. Accountability through elections is an obvious factor; however, legitimacy may be sought either through democratic processes or in other ways, such as strong propaganda.

Here, we set out some of the challenges likely to face emergency management under the three levels developed earlier of routine, non-routine and complex unbounded events.

Routine emergencies

In the West and in many countries with strong institutions, routine emergencies are well handled. There is effective response, a degree of planning and recovery support from both government and non-government sectors. Looking forward, though, these countries may be close to practical limits of capacities in terms of prevention, as well as response, although there are always opportunities for prevention through evolving technology and changing priorities and social values.

However, for many people around the world, emergency management (including response for events widely considered routine) is limited at best. Although this situation is seen most in locations with weak institutions, or which are poor, it is also found in parts of otherwise rich countries. The need here is for the establishment and maintenance of effective emergency management institutions, the general features of which are well known from the experience of comparable countries with better institutional development.

Non-routine emergencies

The situation for non-routine emergencies is generally similar to that for routine emergencies, with some important differences. Since such emergencies are far less frequent than routine events, relevant aspects of emergency management may be relatively neglected compared with those for the more routine. Planning and prevention will typically require cooperation across agencies in order to be effective. This can be said for routine emergencies, too; but with such lower magnitude occurrence, single-agency management is often adequate, even if not ideal.

In non-routine events, the limits of response capacity will frequently be rapidly reached in an environment where spare capacity, whether for monitoring safety regulations or for handling casualties, is seen as inefficient and wasteful. An institutional capacity to harness all aspects of government and non-government resources may be the key to achieving results, including with prevention and preparedness activities. Prevention, for example, will often require active participation from a range of agencies and sectors outside the traditional emergency management mainstream, and will frequently intersect with the institutions of the law and economy, both to remove impediments and to draw on the policy instruments and coercive or incentive capacities that these institutions provide.

Very large-scale non-routine events will merge with some of the characteristics of complex unbounded emergencies – for example, intensive media and political interest and the associated large flows of aid. Such attention is likely to increase with the still-expanding global reach of live media. Even though the attention brings its own problems, lack of interest makes it more difficult for emergency management to justify its efforts and to maintain its resources and capacities between events.

Complex unbounded events

Almost by definition, planning, preparedness and anticipatory approaches will be inadequate, critical resources will be in short supply and political sensitivity will be heightened. Being a rich democracy is no guarantee of successful management for complex unbounded emergencies. Countries and regions may be very wealthy, but lack the institutions needed for management of complex or even otherwise simple but large-scale emergencies.

Perhaps paradoxically, such events often attract intense international media coverage and international, governmental, NGO and individual support, reducing the need to rely largely on local institutional capacity. This is particularly the case for response and some aspects of recovery. It may be far from perfect; but arguably the internationalization of emergency management is one approach to dealing with inadequate local institutional capacity and with the problems posed by exceptionally large and complex events. This is not to downplay efforts to build local capacity, which is needed most for routine emergencies – local capacity by definition will almost always be inadequate in the face of a complex, unbounded disaster. There may be limits to the strategy of internationalization, however, including 'donor fatigue' and an increasing demand for the development of local capacity after repeated calls for assistance, whether in the same jurisdiction or not. Positively, these limits can perhaps be turned into a driver for the large-scale human development agenda needed to attend the gross inequities, poverty and lack of livelihood security that exist in too many parts of the world.

Further challenges are thinking ahead, decision-making in a complex environment full of uncertainties, and the harnessing of resources from across society and internationally for recovery. In preparation, and to reduce the impact of such emergencies, the challenge is to build resilient institutions, organizations and communities, while accepting that anticipatory approaches are of most value for problems that are foreseen and well defined.

International and regional leadership

The international dimension has long been the province of NGOs such as Oxfam, the Red Cross/Crescent Societies and now multilateral agencies led by the United Nations International Strategy for Disaster Reduction and the World Bank's new Global Facility for Disaster Reduction and Recovery, as well as many other groups, prominent or low profile, and active at all phases of emergency management. However, prevention and preparedness continue to receive relatively limited attention despite rhetoric regarding sustainable livelihoods. Redressing this imbalance remains a major challenge. One hopeful sign is the effort devoted to installing warning systems following the Asian tsunami under UN auspices, with leadership provided by former US presidents Bill Clinton and George Bush senior. Some argue that this money would be better spent elsewhere; nevertheless, it shows what can be achieved through strong leadership, utilizing the window of policy opportunity following a major disaster.

Global-level support of this kind is high profile and well resourced. There is much opportunity for increased involvement of neighbouring countries, rather than from distant agencies in every aspect of emergency management. Land borders invite cross-jurisdictional emergencies. More emphasis on regional support and cooperation is emerging and is logical, at least from the perspectives of geography, shared history and tradition, problems and logistics. Some of the vignettes in Chapter 1 illustrate this: the Asian tsunami, flooding in Mozambique and refugees in Goma. Formal and informal arrangements exist in Europe (including by utility companies) and are now part of the agenda at heads of government meetings in Asia and the Pacific.

Prospects: Anticipation, resilience and adaptation

Waiting for disasters to happen is a discredited policy stance; but the alternatives are not easy. Anticipatory approaches are only easily justified and widely accepted provided the form of disaster anticipated is credible. Adaptation as used here is a broader concept since it is not necessarily deliberate in the sense of adaptation to an anticipated problem. It is about adaptation to changed circumstances or sudden disruptions, including increased uncertainty and the likelihood of more challenges for emergency management. This is similar to our definition of resilience, including the ideas of equity, failsafe measures, government intervention, institutional capacity and so on.

Besides the many policy and institutional issues, there are the overarching twin challenges that have recurred throughout this book, which state that disasters:

1   pose whole-of-government and whole-of-society integration problems;
2   demand a greater focus on resilience and cannot be properly addressed through reliance on response.

These are already occurring as shifts in thinking and practice in emergency management; and it has been one purpose of this book to show the extent of the task remaining, especially the policy and institutional, rather than operational, aspects.

Resilience needs to be approached in a realistic fashion by focusing on the people and their fundamental needs – for example, if people do not have food security or a reliable income source (and much of humanity does not), then these issues are likely to be their first priorities in building resilience (Smith and Armstrong, 2006). Clearly, a credible shift towards a stronger resilience/institutional policy style is likely to be deeply political. It concerns who gets what and the role of government in allocating resources across sectors for such issues as water, housing, infrastructure, healthcare and employment.

All policy is *political*, especially strategic policy addressing great differences in vulnerability. In the book, we have stressed this, and it is best for all involved to confront and debate this premise, rather than to pretend it is not so. Doing so without compromising the professionalism and capacity of operational emergency management is the difficulty. The distributive politics of disaster policy are apparent in the tragic aftermath: some people are vulnerable, others are not; some people access recovery resources, others do not. It follows that seeking to reduce vulnerability – the end goal of disaster policy – is also political and, hence, about the institutions of society and strategic policy. If that is more widely accepted and acted on, then emergencies and disasters will have been 'mainstreamed' a little more, and this book will have made a small contribution.

References

Alexander, E. R. (1986) *Approaches to Planning: Introducing Current Planning Theories, Concepts and Issues.* New York: Gordon and Breach Science Publishers

Arnstein, S. (1969) 'A ladder of citizen participation'. *Journal of the American Institute of Planners* **35**: 216–224

Bah, A. and Goodwin, H. (2003) 'Improving access for the informal sector to tourism in The Gambia'. *Pro Poor Tourism (PPT) Working Paper No 15.* London: Economic and Social Research Unit (ESCOR), UK Department for International Development (DFID)

BBC (2002) 'Looting and chaos follow Congo eruption', 18 January 2002, http://news.bbc.co.uk/1/hi/world/africa/1767789.stm

Beck, U. (1992) *Risk Society – Towards a New Modernity.* London: Thousand Oaks; New Delhi: Sage

Bell, M. L. and Davis, D. L. (2001) 'Reassessment of the lethal London fog of 1952: Novel indicators of acute and chronic consequences of acute exposure to air pollution'. *Environmental Health Perspectives* **109** (Supplement): 389–394

Bennett, C. J. and Howlett, M. (1992) 'The lessons of learning: Reconciling theories of policy learning and policy change'. *Policy Sciences* **25**: 275–294

Benson, C. and Clay, E. (2004) *Understanding the Economic and Financial Impacts of Natural Disasters.* Washington, DC: World Bank

Berkhout, F., Leach, M. and Scoones, I. (eds) (2002) *Negotiating Environmental Change: New Perspectives from the Social Sciences.* Cheltenham: Edward Elgar

Bier, V. M. (2001) 'On the state of the art: Risk communication to the public'. *Reliability Engineering and System Safety* **71**: 139–150

Boin, A., Hart, P., Stern, E. and Sundelius, B. (2005) *The Politics of Crisis Management: Public Leadership under Pressure.* Cambridge: Cambridge University Press

Boyden, S. (1987) *Western Civilization in Biological Perspective: Patterns in Biohistory.* Oxford: Clarendon Press

Braithwaite, J. and Drahos, P. (2000) *Global Business Regulation.* Cambridge: Cambridge University Press

Bridgeman, P. and Davis, G. (2001) *The Australian Policy Handbook.* Sydney: Allen and Unwin

Brimblecombe, P. (1987) *The Big Smoke: A History of Air Pollution in London.* London: Methuen

Burby, R. J. and Dalton, L. C. (1994) 'Plans can matter! The role of land use plans and state planning mandates in limiting the development of hazardous areas'. *Public Administration Review* **54**: 229–238

Bye, P. and Horner, M. (1998) *Easter Floods: Volume 1: Report by the Independent Review Team to the Board of the Environment Agency*. Bristol: Environment Agency

CEPAL and BID (Economic Commission for Latin America and the Caribbean and Inter-American Development Bank) (2000) *A Matter of Development: How To Reduce Vulnerability in the Face of Natural Disasters*. CEPAL, Mexico

CIEL (Centre for International Environmental Law) (2007) *Climate Change Program*, www.ciel.org/Climate/programclimate.html

Connor, R. and Dovers, S. (2004) *Institutional Change for Sustainable Development*. Cheltenham: Edward Elgar

Cuny, F. C. (1983) *Disasters and Development*. New York: Oxford University Press

Davis, D. L. (2002) *When Smoke Ran Like Water*. New York: Basic Books

Davis, G., Wanna, J., Warhurst, J. and Weller, P. (1993) *Public Policy in Australia*. Sydney: Allen and Unwin

Dery, D. (1984) *Problem Definition in Policy Analysis*. Lawrence: University of Kansas Press

Dobson, A. (2003) *Citizenship and the Environment*. Oxford: Oxford University Press

Doogan, M. (2006) *The Canberra Fire Storm: Inquest and Enquiry into Four Deaths and Four Fires between 8 and 18 January 2003*. Canberra: ACT Coroners Office

Dovers, S. (1995) 'A framework for scaling and framing policy problems in sustainability'. *Ecological Economics* **12**: 93–106

Dovers, S. (1997) 'Sustainability: demands on policy'. *Journal of Public Policy* **16**: 303–318

Dovers, S. (2004) 'Sustainability and disaster management'. *Australian Journal of Emergency Management* **19(1)**: 21–25

Dovers, S. (2005) *Environment and Sustainability Policy: Creation, Implementation, Evaluation*. Sydney: The Federation Press

Dovers, S. and Handmer, J. W. (1995) 'Ignorance, the precautionary principle and sustainability', *Ambio,* **24**: 92–97

Drabek, T. E. and Hoetmer, G. J. (eds) (1991) *Emergency Management: Principles and Practice for Local Government*. Washington DC: International City Management Association

Dryzek, J. (1996) 'The informal logic of institutional design'. In Goodin, R. E. (ed) *The Theory of Institutional Design*. Cambridge: Cambridge University Press

Dryzek, J. (1997) *The Politics of the Earth: Environmental Discourses*. Oxford: Oxford University Press

Dryzek, J. (2000) *Deliberative Democracy and Beyond: Liberals, Critics, Contestations*. Oxford: Oxford University Press

Dye, T. R. (1983) *Understanding Public Policy*. Englewood Cliffs, NJ: Prentice-Hall

Egeland, J. (2006) *Disaster Risk Reduction: A Call for Engagement*. New York: United Nations, 10 October 2006

Elliott, L. (2005) *Global Politics of the Environment,* 2nd edition. Hampshire: Palgrave Macmillan

EMA (Emergency Management Australia) (1999) *Flood Warning: An Australian Guide.* 2nd edn. Canberra: Emergency Management Australia. (written by Jim Elliott, John Handmer, Chas Keys and John Salter)

EMA (Emergency Management Australia) (2000) *Emergency Risk Management Applications Guide: Australian Emergency Manuals Series, Part II. Approaches to Emergency Management. Volume I – Risk Management.* Canberra: EMA

Erikson, K. T. (1976) *Everything in Its Path: Destruction of Community at Buffalo Creek.* New York: Simon and Schuster

Erikson, K. T. (1979) *In the Wake of the Flood.* London: George Allen and Unwin

Etzioni, A. (1967) 'Mixed scanning: A third approach to decision-making'. *Public Administration Review* 27: 385–392

European Environment Agency (2001) *Late Lessons from Early Warnings: The Precautionary Principle 1886–2000.* Copenhagen: European Environment Agency

Finer, S. E. (1997) *The History of Government from the Earliest Times.* Oxford: Oxford University Press

Fischer, F. (2003) *Reframing Public Policy: Discursive Politics and Deliberative Practices.* Oxford: Oxford University Press

Fritz. C. (1961) 'Disaster'. In Merton, R. K. and Nisbet, R. A. (eds) *Contemporary Social Problems.* New York: Harcourt Press, pp651–694

Foresight (2004) *Foresight Future Flooding.* London: Office of Science and Technology

Fung, A. and Wright, E. O. (eds) (2003) *Deepening Democracy: Institutional Innovation in Empowered Participatory Governance.* London: Verso

Funtowicz, S. O. and Ravetz, J. R. (1993) 'Science for the post-normal age'. *Futures* 25: 739–755

Giddens, A. (2000) *The Third Way and Its Critics.* Cambridge: Polity Press

Gillroy, J. M. and Wade, M. (eds) (1992) *The Moral Dimensions of Public Policy Choice: Beyond the Market Paradigm.* Pittsburgh: University of Pittsburgh Press

Goodin, R. E. (1996) 'Institutions and their design'. In Goodin, R. E. (ed) *The Theory of Institutional Design.* Cambridge: Cambridge University Press, pp1–53

Gunningham, N. and Grabosky, P. (1999) *Smart Regulation: Designing Environmental Policy.* Oxford: Clarendon Press

Handmer, J. W. (1986) 'Flood policy reversal in NSW'. *Disasters* 9(4): 279–285

Handmer, J. (2000) 'Are flood warnings futile?' *Australasian Journal of Disaster and Trauma Studies,* 2000-2, www.massey.ac.nz/~trauma/

Handmer, J. (2003a) 'We are all vulnerable'. *Australian Journal of Emergency Management* 18(3): 55–60

Handmer, J. (2003b) 'Adaptive capacity: What does it mean in the context of natural hazards?' in: Smith, J. B., Klein, R. and Huq, S. (eds) *Climate Change: Adaptive Capacity and Development.* London: Imperial College Press, pp51–70

Handmer, J. (2006) 'American exceptionalism or universal lesson: The implications of Hurricane Katrina for Australia'. *Australian Journal of Emergency Management* 21(1): 29–42

Handmer, J. and Choong, W. (2006) 'Disaster resilience through local economic development'. *Australian Journal of Emergency Management* 21(4): 8–15

Handmer, J. and Dovers, S. (1996) 'A typology of resilience: Rethinking institutions for sustainability'. *Industrial and Environmental Crisis Quarterly* **9**: 482–511

Handmer, J., Loh, E. and Choong, W. (2007) 'Using law to address vulnerability to natural disasters'. *Georgetown Journal on Poverty Law and Policy* **XIV(I)**: 13–38

Handmer, J. and Monson, R. (2004) 'Does a rights based approach make a difference? The role of public law in vulnerability reduction'. *International Journal of Mass Emergencies and Disasters* **22(3)**: 43–59

Handmer, J. and Proudley, B. (2005) *The Science of Surprise: Implementing Post-Normal Science for Managing Complex Unbounded Problems*. Final Report for EMA. Canberra: EMA

Handmer, J. Read, C. and Percovich, O. (2002) *Disaster Loss Assessment Guidelines*. Australia: Qld Department of Emergency Services and Emergency Management Australia

Handmer, J. and Tibbits, A. (2005) 'Is staying at home the safest option during wildfire? Historical evidence for an Australian approach'. *Environmental Hazards* **6**: 81–91

Hart, K., (1973) 'Informal income opportunities and urban employment in Ghana', *The Journal of Modern African Studies* **11(1)**: 61–89

Haynes, K., Barclay, J. and Pidgeon, N. (in press) 'Blame and conspiracy: Factors influencing risk communication during a volcanic crisis'. *Bulletin of Volcanology*

Healey, P. (1997) *Collaborative Planning: Shaping Places in Fragmented Societies*. London: Macmillan

Herrington, J. (1989) *Planning Processes: An Introduction for Geographers*. Cambridge: Cambridge University Press

Hezri, A. A. (2004) 'Sustainability indicators system and policy processes in Malaysia: A framework for utilization and learning'. *Journal of Environmental Management* **73**: 357–371

Hogwood, B. W. and Gunn, L. A. (1984) *Policy Analysis for the Real World*. Oxford: Oxford University Press

Holling, C. S. (1978) *Adaptive Environmental Management and Assessment*. Chichester: Wiley

Honadle, B. W. (1981) 'A capacity-building framework: A search for concept and purpose'. *Public Administration Review* **September/October**: 575–580

Hood, C. and Jackson, M. (1992) 'The new public management: A recipe for disaster?' in Parker, D. J. and Handmer, J. (eds) *Hazard Management and Emergency Planning*. London: James and James, pp109–125

Hopkins, A. (2000) *Lessons from Longford: The Esso Gas Plant Explosion*. Sydney: CCH Australia

Hopkins, A. (2005) *Safety, Culture and Risk: The Organizational Causes of Disasters*. Sydney: CCH Australia

Howlett, M. (1991) 'Policy instruments, policy styles, and policy implementation: National approaches to theories of instrument choice'. *Policy Studies Journal* **19**: 1–21

Howlett, M. (1998) 'Predictable and unpredictable policy windows: Institutional and exogenous correlates of Canadian Federal agenda-setting'. *Canadian Journal of Political Science* **31**: 495–524

Howlett, M. and Ramesh, M. (2003) *Studying Public Policy: Policy Cycles and Policy Subsystems*. Don Mills, Ontario: Oxford University Press

IFRC (International Federation of Red Cross and Red Crescent Societies) (2001) *World Disasters Report 2001*. Geneva: IFRC

IPCC (Intergovernmental Panel on Climate Change) (2007) *Climate Change 2007: The Physical Science Basis*. Contribution of Working Group I to the Fourth Assessment Report (AR4), Summary for Policymakers. Geneva: IPCC

Irwin, A. (1995) *Citizen Science: A Study of People, Expertise and Sustainable Development*. London: Routledge

Jaquemet, I. (2001) 'Post-flood recovery in Viet Nam' in *World Disasters Report 2001*. Geneva: IFRC, Chapter 5

Jasanoff, S., Markle, G., Petersen, J. and Pinch, T. (eds) (1995) *Handbook of Science and Technology Studies*. London and New Dehli: Sage

Jenkins-Smith, H. and Sabatier, P. (1994) 'Evaluating the advocacy coalition framework'. *Journal of Public Policy* 14: 175–203

Kingdon, J. W. (1984) *Agendas, Alternatives and Public Policy*. Boston: Little, Brown

Lafferty, W. M. and Meadowcroft, J. (eds) (2000) *Implementing Sustainable Development*. Oxford: Oxford University Press

Lasswell, H. (1951) 'The policy orientation'. In Lerner, D. and Lasswell, H. (eds) *The Policy Sciences: Recent Developments in Scope and Methods*. Stanford: Stanford University Press, pp3–15

Laswell, H. (1971) *A Pre-View of the Policy Sciences*. New York: Elsevier

Lee, K. N. (1993) *Compass and Gyroscope: Integrating Science and Politics for the Environment*. Washington, DC: Island Press

Leeuw, F. L., Rist, R. C. and Sonnichsen, R. C. (eds) (1994) *Can Governments Learn? Comparative Perspectives on Evaluation and Organizational Learning*. New Brunswick, NJ: Transaction Publishers

Levy, B. S. and Sidel, V. W. (2000) *War and Public Health*. Washington, DC: American Public Health Association

Lindblom, C. E. (1959) 'The science of muddling through'. *Public Administration Review* 19: 79–88

Lindblom, C. E. (1979) 'Still muddling, not yet through'. *Public Administration Review* 39: 517–526

Lindblom, C. E. and Cohen, D. K. (1979) *Usable Knowledge: Social Science and Social Problem Solving*. New Haven: Yale University Press

Linder, S. H. and Peters, B. G. (1989) 'Instruments of government: Perceptions and contexts'. *Journal of Public Policy* 9: 35–58

Lynn, K. (2003) 'Wildfire and rural poverty'. *Natural Hazards Observer* **November XXIX(2)**: 10–11

March, J. G. and Olsen, J. P. (1979) *Ambiguity and Choice in Organizations*. Bergen: Universitetsforlaget

Marine Accident Investigation Branch (undated) *Herald of Free Enterprise Report*. London: Marine Accident Investigation Branch, UK Department of Transport

May, P. (1992) 'Policy learning and policy failure'. *Journal of Public Policy* **12**: 331–354

May, P., Burby, R. J., Ericksen, N. J., Handmer, J., Dixon, J. E., Michaels, S. and Smith, D. I. (1996) *Environmental Management and Governance: Intergovernmental Approaches to Hazards and Sustainability*. London: Routledge

May, P. and Handmer, J. (1992) 'Regulatory policy design: Cooperative versus deterrent mandates'. *Australian Journal of Public Administration* **511**: 43–53

McArthur, A. G. and Cheney, N. P. (1967) *Report on the Southern Tasmanian Bushfires of 7 February 1967*. Hobart: Forestry Commission Tasmania, Government Printer

McGurk, T. (2005) 'Marketing a monopoly (Merseyside Fire Service)'. Keynote address presented at *AFAC/Bushfire CRC 2005 Conference*, Auckland

McLaughlin, K., Osborne, S. P. and Ferlie, E. (eds) (2002) *New Public Management: Current Trends and Future Prospects*. Routledge: London

McLean, I. and Johnes, M. (2000) *Aberfan: Government and Disasters*. Cardiff: Welsh Academic Press

Mileti, D. (1999) *Disasters by Design: A Reassessment of Natural Hazards in the United States*. Washington, DC: Joseph Henry Press

Mitchell, J. K. (1999) *Crucibles of Disaster: Megacities and disasters in transition*. Tokyo: United Nations University Press

Munich Re (2006) *Topics Geo: Natural Catastrophes 2006 Analysis, Assessment, Positions*, Munich Re, www.munichre.com/publications

Munton, R. (2002) 'Deliberative democracy and environmental decision-making'. In Berkhout, F., Leach, M. and Scoones, I. (eds) *Negotiating Environmental Change: New Perspectives from the Social Sciences*. Cheltenham: Edward Elgar

Newell, B. and Wasson, R. (2002) 'Social system vs solar system: Why policy makers need history' in Castelein, S. and Otte, A. (eds) *Conflict and Cooperation Related to International Water Resources: Historical Perspectives*. Paris: UNESCO, pp3–17

North, D. C. (1990) *Institutions, Institutional Change and Economic Performance*. Cambridge: Cambridge University Press

NSW (New South Wales) (2001) *Floodplain Management Manual: The Management of Flood Liable Land*. Sydney: NSW Government

OECD (Organisation for Economic Co-operation and Development) and Pourtier, R. (2003) *Central Africa and the Cross Border Regions: Reconstruction and Integration Projects*, Study produced for Initiative for Central Africa (INICA). Paris: OECD, June 2003.

O'Keefe, P., Westgate, K. and Wisner, B. (1976) 'Taking the naturalness out of natural disasters'. *Nature* **260**: 566–567

Oxfam (2002) www.oxfam.ca/news/Congo/Update_Jan21.htm

Patton, M. Q. (1997) *Utilisation-Focused Evaluation: The New Century Text*. Thousand Oaks, CL: Sage Publications

Patton, M. (2002) *Qualitative Research and Evaluation Methods*. Thousand Oaks, CL: Sage Publications

Pelling, M. (2003) *The Vulnerability of Cities: Natural Disasters and Social Resilience*. London: Earthscan

Perrow, C. (1984) *Normal Accidents: Living with High-Risk Technologies*. New York: Basic Books

Peters, B. G. and Pierre, J. (2003) *Handbook of Public Administration*. London: Sage Publications

Pidgeon, N., Kasperson R. E. and Slovic, P. (2003) *The Social Amplification of Risk*. Cambridge: Cambridge University Press

Pierre, J. and Peters, B. G. (2000) *Governance, Politics and the State*. New York: Macmillan

Quarantelli, E. L. (ed) (1998) *What Is a Disaster? Perspectives on the Question*. London: Routledge

Reichhardt, T., Check, E. and Marris, E. (2005) 'After the flood – special report'. *Nature* 8 September, **437**: 174–176

Rhodes, R. A. W., Binder, S. A. and Roderman, B. A. (eds) (2006) *The Oxford Handbook of Political Institutions*. Oxford: Oxford University Press

Rodriguez, H., Quarantelli, E. and Dynes, R. (2006) *Handbook of Disaster Research*. New York: Springer Sociology

Rose, R. (2005) *Learning from Comparative Public Policy: A Practical Guide*. London: Routledge

Rossi, P. and Freeman, H. (1993) *Evaluation: A Systematic Approach*. Newbury Park: Sage Publications

RUSI (Royal United Services Institute for Defence and Security Studies) (2007) *Climate Change: The Global Security Impact*. Conference at RUSI, London, 24 January, www.rusi.org

Salamon, L. M. and Elliott, O. V. (2002) *The Tools of Government: A Guide to the New Governance*. Oxford: Oxford University Press

Smith, D. J. and Armstrong, S. (2006) *If the World Were a Village*. London: A&C Black

Smithson, M. (1989) *Ignorance and Uncertainty: Emerging Paradigms*. New York: Springer-Verlag

Smithson, M. (1991) 'The changing nature of ignorance'. In Handmer, J., Dutton, B., Guerin, B. and Smithson, M. (eds) *New Perspectives on Uncertainty and Risk*. Mt Macedon: CRES Australian National University and Australian Counter Disaster College

Sparrow, J. (2001) 'Relief, recovery and root causes'. *World Disasters Report 2001*. Geneva: IFRC, Chapter 1

Stallings, R. A. (2002) *Methods of Disaster Research*. Philadelphia: Xlibris (Random House)

Standards Australia (2004) *Australian Standard/New Zealand Standard 4360-2004: Risk Management*. Sydney: Standards Australia

Steffen, W., Sanderson, A., Tyson, P., Jäger, J., Matson, P., Moore III, B., Oldfield, F., Richardson, K., Schellnhuber, H. J., Turner II, B. L. and Wasson, R. (2004) *Global Change and the Earth System: A Planet under Pressure*. Berlin, Heidelburg, New York: Springer-Verlag

Stern, N. (2006) *The Economics of Climate Change: The Stern Review*. Cambridge: Cambridge University Press

Stiglitz, J. E. (2002*) Globalization and Its Discontents*. London: Penguin

Tarrant, M. (2006) Pers comm, Emergency Management Australia, Mt Macedon, June 2006

Tuan, Y. F. (1979) *Landscapes of Fear*. New York: Pantheon

Turner, B. (1978) *Man-Made Disasters*. London: Wykeham

Turner, B. and Pidgeon, N. (1997) *Man-Made Disasters*, second edition. London: Butterworth

Twigg, J. (2004) 'Education, information, communications'. In *Disaster Risk Reduction: Mitigation and Preparedness in Development and Emergency Programming*. Good Practice Review No 9. London: Humanitarian Practice Network, Chapter 11, pp165–195

UNDP (United Nations Development Programme) (2005) *Fast Facts: The Faces of Poverty*, UN Millennium Project, http://mirror.undp.org/unmillenniumproject/facts/index.htm

UN–ISDR (United Nations International Strategy for Disaster Reduction) (1999) *Declaration of International Strategy for Disaster Reduction*. Geneva: UN Office of Humanitarian Affairs

UN–ISDR (2004) *Hyogo Framework for Disaster Prevention*. Geneva: ISDR

UN–ISDR (2005) *Know Risk*. Leicester, UK: Tudor House

US Center for Naval Analysis (2007) *National Security and the Threat of Climate Change*. Alexandria, VA: CNA Corporation

US Committee for Refugees (2000) *World Refugee Survey 2000*. Washington, DC: US Committee for Refugees

US National Science and Technology Council (2005) *Grand Challenges for Disaster Reduction*. Subcommittee on Disaster Reduction. Washington, DC: Executive Office of the President of the United States

van der Grijp, N. and Olsthoorn, X. (2000) *Institutional Framework for the Management of the Rivers Rhine and Meuse in The Netherlands: An Overview*. Report no D-00/03. Amsterdam: Institute for Environmental Studies, Vrije University

van Duin, M. J., Bezuyen, M. J. and Rosenthal, U. (1995) *Evacuaties bij hoog water: Zelfredzaamheid en overheidszorg [Evacuation Due to Flooding: Private Action and Government Care]*. Leiden and Rotterdam: Crisis Research Team, Leiden University and Erasmus University

Walter, J. (2001) 'Disaster data: Key trends and statistics' in *World Disaster Report 2001: Focus on Recovery*. Geneva: ICRC, Chapter 8

White, G. F. (1945) *Human Adjustments to Floods*. Chicago, IL: University of Chicago Press

Wholey, J. S., Hatry, H. P. and Newcomer, K. P. (2004) *Handbook of Practical Program Evaluation*. San Francisco: Jossey-Bass

Wisner, B., Blaikie, P., Cannon, T. and Davis, I. (2004) *At Risk: Natural Hazards, People's Vulnerability and Disasters*. 2nd ed. London: Routledge

Wynne, B. (1993) 'Uncertainty and environmental learning', in Jackson, T. (ed) *Clean Production Strategies: Developing Preventive Environmental Management in the Industrial Economy*. Boca Ratan: Lewis Publishers

Index